Elisabeth Rakus-Andersson

Fuzzy and Rough Techniques in Medical Diagnosis and Medication

Studies in Fuzziness and Soft Computing, Volume 212

**Editor-in-chief**
Prof. Janusz Kacprzyk
Systems Research Institute
Polish Academy of Sciences
ul. Newelska 6
01-447 Warsaw
Poland
E-mail: kacprzyk@ibspan.waw.pl

---

Further volumes of this series can be found on our homepage: springer.com

Vol. 196. James J. Buckley
*Fuzzy Probability and Statistics,* 2006
ISBN 978-3-540-30841-6

Vol. 197. Enrique Herrera-Viedma, Gabriella Pasi, Fabio Crestani (Eds.)
*Soft Computing in Web Information Retrieval,* 2006
ISBN 978-3-540-31588-9

Vol. 198. Hung T. Nguyen, Berlin Wu
*Fundamentals of Statistics with Fuzzy Data,* 2006
ISBN 978-3-540-31695-4

Vol. 199. Zhong Li
*Fuzzy Chaotic Systems,* 2006
ISBN 978-3-540-33220-6

Vol. 200. Kai Michels, Frank Klawonn, Rudolf Kruse, Andreas Nürnberger
*Fuzzy Control,* 2006
ISBN 978-3-540-31765-4

Vol. 201. Cengiz Kahraman (Ed.)
*Fuzzy Applications in Industrial Engineering,* 2006
ISBN 978-3-540-33516-0

Vol. 202. Patrick Doherty, Witold Łukaszewicz, Andrzej Skowron, Andrzej Szałas
*Knowledge Representation Techniques: A Rough Set Approach,* 2006
ISBN 978-3-540-33518-4

Vol. 203. Gloria Bordogna, Giuseppe Psaila (Eds.)
*Flexible Databases Supporting Imprecision and Uncertainty,* 2006
ISBN 978-3-540-33288-6

Vol. 204. Zongmin Ma (Ed.)
*Soft Computing in Ontologies and Semantic Web,* 2006
ISBN 978-3-540-33472-9

Vol. 205. Mika Sato-Ilic, Lakhmi C. Jain
*Innovations in Fuzzy Clustering,* 2006
ISBN 978-3-540-34356-1

Vol. 206. A. Sengupta (Ed.)
*Chaos, Nonlinearity, Complexity,* 2006
ISBN 978-3-540-31756-2

Vol. 207. Isabelle Guyon, Steve Gunn, Masoud Nikravesh, Lotfi A. Zadeh (Eds.)
*Feature Extraction,* 2006
ISBN 978-3-540-35487-1

Vol. 208. Oscar Castillo, Patricia Melin, Janusz Kacprzyk, Witold Pedrycz (Eds.)
*Hybrid Intelligent Systems,* 2007
ISBN 978-3-540-37419-0

Vol. 209. Alexander Mehler, Reinhard Köhler
*Aspects of Automatic Text Analysis,* 2007
ISBN 978-3-540-37520-3

Vol. 210. Mike Nachtegael, Dietrich Van der Weken, Etienne E. Kerre, Wilfried Philips (Eds.)
*Soft Computing in Image Processing,* 2007
ISBN 978-3-540-38232-4

Vol. 211. Alexander Gegov
*Complexity Management in Fuzzy Systems,* 2007
ISBN 978-3-540-38883-8

Vol. 212. Elisabeth Rakus-Andersson
*Fuzzy and Rough Techniques in Medical Diagnosis and Medication,* 2007
ISBN 978-3-540-49707-3

Elisabeth Rakus-Andersson

# Fuzzy and Rough Techniques in Medical Diagnosis and Medication

Springer

Elisabeth Rakus-Andersson
Docent in Mathematics
Blekinge Institute of Technology
Department of Mathematics and Science
37179 Karlskrona
Sweden
E-mail: Elisabeth.Andersson@bth.se

Library of Congress Control Number: 2006937349

ISSN print edition: 1434-9922
ISSN electronic edition: 1860-0808
ISBN-10 3-540-49707-2 Springer Berlin Heidelberg New York
ISBN-13 978-3-540-49707-3 Springer Berlin Heidelberg New York



Springer is a part of Springer Science+Business Media
springer.com


Typesetting: by the author and techbooks using a Springer LaTeX macro package
Cover design: Erich Kirchner, Heidelberg

Printed on acid-free paper SPIN: 11940234 89/techbooks 5 4 3 2 1 0

To Irena and Christer

# Contents

**List of Figures** .......... **IX**

**List of Tables** .......... **XI**

**1 Introduction** .......... **1**

**2 Fundamental Items** .......... **3**
2.1 Introduction .......... 3
2.2 Fuzzy Sets .......... 4
2.3 Basic Operations on Fuzzy Sets .......... 12
2.4 Linguistic Variables .......... 19
2.5 Fuzzy Relations .......... 23

**3 Medical Diagnosis** .......... **31**
3.1 Introduction .......... 31
3.2 The Modus Ponens Law in Medical Diagnosis .......... 31
3.3 The *Patient – Symptom* Relation .......... 33
3.3.1 Simple Qualitative Biological Parameters .......... 33
3.3.2 Compound Qualitative Biological Features .......... 34
3.3.3 Compound Quantitative Biological Features .......... 40
3.4 The *Symptom – Diagnosis* Relation .......... 45
3.4.1 Numerical Representations of Linguistic Variables .......... 46
3.4.2 Relations of "*Presence*" and "*Decisive Character*" .......... 52
3.5 The *Patient – Diagnosis* Relation .......... 55

**4 Complementary Solutions in Diagnostic Models** .......... **63**
4.1 Introduction .......... 63
4.2 OWA Operators in Decision Relations .......... 63
4.3 Fuzzy Set Distances in Diagnostic Decisions .......... 71
4.4 Diagnostic Processes Extended in Time Intervals .......... 80
4.5 Rough Set Theory in the Classification of Diagnoses .......... 87

**5 Evaluation of Medicine Action Levels** .......... **93**
5.1 Introduction .......... 93
5.2 Theoretical Assumptions of Eigen Fuzzy Problem .......... 93
5.3 Eigen Sets in Medicine Effectiveness Levels .......... 100

5.4 Order Operations on Fuzzy Numbers ... 104
5.5 Eigen Fuzzy Sets with Fuzzy Numbers ... 114
5.6 The *L-R* Fuzzy Numbers as Drug Efficiency Intervals ... 119

**6 The Choice of Optimal Medicines ... 127**
6.1 Introduction ... 127
6.2 Fuzzy Utilities in Decision-Making Models ... 127
6.2.1 Jain's Utility Matrix as the *Drug – Symptom* Table ... 128
6.2.2 The Solution of Jain's Decision Case ... 134
6.3 Group Decision-Making in the Selection of Drugs ... 140
6.4 Unequal Objectives in the Choice of Medicines ... 144
6.4.1 The Design of Objectives-Constraints ... 145
6.4.2 The Power-Importance of Objectives ... 148
6.4.3 Minimization of Regret ... 151

**7 Approximation of Clock-like Point Sets ... 155**
7.1 Introduction ... 155
7.2 Fitting of $\pi$-functions to Clock-like Polygons ... 155
7.3 Rough Sets in Classifying of Clock-like Polygons ... 165
7.4 *s*-functions in Fitting to Letter-shaped Polygons ... 168
7.5 The Classification of Letter-shaped Polygons ... 179

**References ... 183**

**Index ... 189**

# List of Figures


2.1 The characteristic function of the crisp set $C = [4, 8]$ ........................ 4
2.2 Fuzzy set $A = \{(x, \mu_A(x))\}, x \in [0, 10]$ ........................ 6
2.3 The continuous fuzzy set "*young*" ........................ 7
2.4 The function $s(x, 25, 37.5, 50)$ ........................ 8
2.5 The membership function of the set "*young*" as the *s*-class function ....... 9
2.6 The function $\pi(x,20,45)$ ........................ 10
2.7 The fuzzy sets "*young*", "*middle-aged*" and "*old*" in $X = [0, 100]$ ......... 11
2.8 The membership function of the set "*body temperature*" ........................ 12
2.9 The union of fuzzy sets $A$ and $B$ from Ex. 2.10 ........................ 13
2.10 The intersection of $A$ and $B$ from Ex. 2.10 ........................ 14
2.11 The complement of the set $B$ from Ex. 2.10 ........................ 15
2.12 The membership function of the set "*young or experienced*" ........................ 16
2.13 The membership function of the set "*young and experienced*" ........................ 17
2.14 The constraint $R$("*often*") over the reference set $A = [0, 100]$ ........................ 21
2.15 The fuzzy constraints of terms representing "*presence of S in D*" ......... 22
2.16 "*A strong and proportional construction of the man's body*" ........................ 25

3.1 The membership function of the compound qualitative symptom $S_j$ ...... 37
3.2 The membership function of the symptom $S_8$ ........................ 42
3.3 The membership function of the symptom $S_8$ with modifications ......... 43
3.4 The membership functions of fuzzy variables generated by "*seldom*" .... 49
3.5 The membership functions of fuzzy variables generated by "*often*" ...... 50
3.6 The terms from the lists "*presence*" and "*decisive character*" ........................ 51

4.1 The comparison of sets $PD_3$ and $AP(PD_3)$ for patient $P$ ........................ 73
4.2 The distance between $AP(PD_3)_{D_1}$ and $AP(PD_3)$ ........................ 74
4.3 The distance between $AP(PD_3)_{D_3}$ and $AP(PD_3)$ ........................ 74
4.4 The comparison between $PD_4$ (or $PD_5$) and $JP(PD_4)$ (or $JP(PD_5)$) ....... 76

5.1 $A \subseteq B$ for $\mu_A(x) = s(x, 30, 50, 70)$ and $\mu_B(x) = s(x, 10, 50, 90)$ ........................ 95
5.2 The fuzzy number $N = (40, 2, 3)$ ........................ 105
5.3 Minimum for $N_1 = (25, 2, 3)$ and $N_2 = (40, 1, 5)$ according to (5.13) .... 106
5.4 Minimum for $N_1 = (40, 2, 3)$ and $N_2 = (42, 1, 5)$ made by (5.14) ......... 107
5.5 Maximum for $N_1 = (25, 2, 3)$ and $N_2 = (40, 1, 5)$ due to (5.15) ........... 108
5.6 Maximum for $N_1 = (40, 2, 3)$ and $N_2 = (42, 1, 5)$ computed by (5.16)... 109
5.7 Minimum for $N_1 = (40, 7, 8)$ and $N_2 = (42, 3, 2)$ as the result of (5.14)..113

5.8 Minimum for $N_1 = (40, 7, 8)$ and $N_2 = (42, 3, 2)$ due to (5.17)........... 114
5.9 The type-1 fuzzy set $B_1 = \{(10, 0.2), (20, 0.3), (30, 0.15)\}$.............. 116
5.10 The type-2 set $B_2 = \{(10, (20, 3, 2)), (20, (30, 5, 7)), (30, (15, 3, 4))\}$... 117
5.11 Terms of drug effectiveness expressed as fuzzy numbers................ 120
5.12 Fuzzy numbers $A(S_1)$, $A(S_2)$, $A(S_3)$ of the eigen set $A$ of the relation $R$.. 126

6.1 The fuzzy constrains $R_1$–$R_{11}$.................................................. 131
6.2 The 0.5-level of $A$ characterized by $\pi(x, 20, 50)$............................ 141
6.3 The set $R_1$ as the directed graph.............................................. 143
6.4 The set $R_{0.83}$ as the directed graph............................................ 143
6.5 The set $R_{0.67}$ as the directed graph............................................ 144

7.1 The polygon reflecting $A = \{(x, y)\}$.......................................... 156
7.2 The polygon representing $A_1$................................................... 157
7.3 The $\pi$-function for $\alpha_1 = 30$, $\gamma_1 = \alpha_2 = 32.5$, $\gamma_2 = 35$ and $\varepsilon = 0.25$......... 159
7.4 The approximation of $A_1$ by the truncated $\pi$-function..................... 162
7.5 The approximation of $A^*$ by truncated $\pi$ functions........................ 163
7.6 The sampled $\pi$ in the approximation of $A$.................................. 165
7.7 $\pi_1$–$\pi_6$ in approximation of polygons $A_1$–$A_6$................................ 167
7.8 The example of a letter-shaped polygon reflecting $A = \{(x, y)\}$.......... 169
7.9 The approximation of $A$ by "sampled truncated $s$"......................... 173
7.10 The approximated polygons $A^1$–$A^5$.......................................... 175
7.11 The curves $A^1$–$A^5$ with their start points at the origin...................... 176
7.12 The curves $A^1$–$A^5$ over the common interval [0, 1]......................... 178

# List of Tables


3.1 The representatives of the variables "*never*", ..., "*always*" ........ 51
3.2 The numerical description of fuzzy variables in "*presence*" ........ 52
3.3 Linguistic frequency and importance of $S_1, \ldots, S_{10}$ in $D_1, D_2, D_3$ ........ 53
3.4 Numerical frequency and importance of $S_1, \ldots, S_{10}$ in $D_1, D_2, D_3$ ........ 54
3.5 $P_1$'s diagnostic decision based on $PD_3$, $PD_4$ and $PD_5$ ........ 59
3.6 $P_2$'s diagnostic decision based on $PD_3$, $PD_4$ and $PD_5$ ........ 60

4.1 Weighted relation compositions in the diagnostic decision ........ 69
4.2 The diagnostic decision concerning patient $P_3$ ........ 79
4.3 The distances $d_k$, $d_k'$ and $d_k''$, $k = 1, 2, 3$, evaluated for patient $P_3$ ........ 80
4.4 The relations $TPD_3$, $TPD_4$ and $TPD_5$ made for $P_1$ ........ 86
4.5 The final acceptance of diagnosis by means of distances ........ 86
4.6 The table $(P, S, D_1)$ in diagnosis classification ........ 90

5.1 Sign configurations for symptoms $S_j$, $S_k$ in $P_1$–$P_7$ ........ 101

6.1 The representatives of linearly modeled effectiveness terms ........ 146

7.1 The relationship between $y$-values and codes ........ 166
7.2 The decision table $I = (U, B, D)$ of clock-like polygons $A_1$–$A_6$ ........ 168
7.3 The decision table $I = (U, B, D)$ for letter-like curves $A^1$–$A^5$ ........ 180

# 1 Introduction

In the late eighties of the twentieth century I encountered a paper referring to mathematics dealing with imprecision applied to medical diagnosis. I was working in the area of medical statistics at that time, and obviously I was interested in the contents of the paper. After I had read it I became fascinated by new possibilities of medical data interpretation and processing proposed by the author. The new world of fuzziness, originated by Professor Lotfi Zadeh, seemed to open up to me and I started reading all accessible material about fuzzy set theory.

Many years have passed since then. We are now living in the information society and we do not experience troubles in reaching scientific material. Lately I have read many papers and books about treating medical tasks solved by using fuzzy ideas. I am still keen on tracing applications in medicine, and by myself I have been contributing to some concepts in this subject that has motivated me to prepare my own book. The objective of writing such a book has been a little particular, namely, I have intended to present the subject of fuzzy tools and techniques in medicine for eventual users. These, maybe representatives of medical or pharmacological staffs, are not expected to possess a large amount of mathematical knowledge. On the contrary, we have a feeling that mathematics is a subject making non-professionally educated specialists almost afraid of meeting comprehensive difficulties. To build a bridge between theoretical, mathematical excerpts and practical applications, I have formed my material as a sequence of occurrences in which a patient appears to be recovered from his or her illness. The patient needs to be diagnosed and treated by effective means to become healthy again. In this way the reader should have an impression that he or she follows the patient and his or her problems.

Therefore I have decided to avoid inserting a large number of mathematical definitions and theorems that have not much meaning in practice. I have only selected formal fuzzy concepts that are needed for medical models. To facilitate the understanding process for a reader, I have added many examples in which even simple operations are thoroughly analyzed. The user can follow the steps of examples without implementing a computer program. As we can expect, the book is not a survey of all theoretical concepts typical of fuzzy sets; such monographs already exist. Nevertheless, some beginners can use it to learn the basics included in fuzzy set theory. In spite of limiting the mathematical dimension, the work should convince the reader of the richness of applicable fuzzy models in natural sciences, especially medicine.

Elisabeth Rakus-Andersson: *Fuzzy and Rough Techniques in Medical Diagnosis and Medication*,
StudFuzz **212**, 1–2 (2007)
www.springerlink.com 

Incidentally, I also discovered the usefulness of rough set theory for the classification of objects. Thus, some rough classification methods are considered as well.

The first part of the book – Chapter 2 – introduces some necessary elements of fuzzy set theory to enable the reader to repeat the processes and interpret imprecise information in further studies. A classical fuzzy diagnostic model with my own extensions is discussed in Chapter 3. Since a diagnostic decision is sometimes not quite clear, I have added Chapter 4 filled with my own contributions to improve informative validity of collected data. The model, presenting the essence of clinical examinations extended throughout time, constitutes one of the supplements.

After stating the right diagnosis the patient needs to be cured. Methods of drug effectiveness measurements are compared in Chapter 5, while a choice of the optimal medicine is made in Chapter 6. The last models are totally based on my own research results. Lastly, the solution of an approximation problem that is of considerable importance for our discussion is suggested in Chapter 7. Many times we obtain very irregular two-dimensional point sets that cannot be approximated by applying them to standard numerical methods. Some fuzzy membership functions have been adopted to provide the sets with smooth curves acting for them as tight envelopes. Even though the method is tested without medical examples, we are able to notice its usefulness in practical tests.

It should be emphasized that all models are also applicable to other fields, especially to technical domains after necessary adaptations.

This book could not have filled its role without professional medical support. I would like to thank Professors in Medicine – Alicja Kurnatowska and Anna Jegier – for a piece of medical advice and simple but illustrative examples.

I am very grateful to the representatives of Springer Verlag and to the series editor Professor Janusz Kacprzyk for giving me a chance to publish this material concerning applicable fuzzy medical models presented from my point of view. I hope that this work can bridge a gap between scientific reports, strictly treating separate domains, and, in this way, interdisciplinary groups of researchers can surely notice that there are prospects of linking theoretical fuzzy tools to practical medical exercises.

Karlskrona – Sweden
July 2006

*Elisabeth Rakus-Andersson*

# 2 Fundamental Items

## 2.1 Introduction

We are still accustomed to our traditional tools of reasoning being strict and precise. In conventional binary logic a statement can be true or false, and there is no place for even a little uncertainty in this judgement. By looking at sets, we can state that an element either belongs to a set or does not. We call these kinds of sets *crisp sets*. In practice we often experience those real situations that are represented by crisp sets, as impossible to describe accurately. If we assign a truth-value of one to the element that is included in the set, and a truth-value comparable to zero to such an element that lies outside the set, we create the range of two-valued logic. This sort of logic assumes that precise symbols must be employed, and it is therefore not applicable to the real existence but only to an imagined existence.

The creator of fuzzy set theory, Lotfi A. Zadeh, referred to the last hypothesis when he wrote: "As the complexity of a system increases, our ability to make precise and yet significant statements about its behaviour diminishes until the threshold is reached beyond which precision and significance become almost mutually exclusive characteristics" [88, 95].

If we consider the characteristic features of real world systems, we will conclude that real situations are very often uncertain or vague in a number of ways. If the information demanded by a system is lacking, the future state of such a system may not be known completely. This type of uncertainty has been handled by probability theories and statistics, and it is called stochastic uncertainty. The vagueness, concerning the description of the semantic meaning of the events, phenomena, or statements themselves, is called fuzziness [95].

Fuzziness can be found in many areas of daily life, especially in medicine. We look for the methods that help us to express the borders of such sets as "*young*", "*middle-aged*", "*old*", "*seldom*", "*rarely*", "*often*", "*high temperature*", "*low sugar level*" and the like. By using the traditional methods we are not able to express exactly the range of a set, e.g., "*young*" when defining the upper limit as, say, 26. Someone can ask "Why not 27?"

Almost every human being cannot be classified as "*totally healthy*" or "*totally ill*" in accordance with the two states of truth assumed by binary logic. It is more so since the conditions of health should be characterized by grades of a scale that propose the many nuances between "*total health*" and "*total sickness*". Thus we introduce the fuzzy apparatus to extend a notion of the set under the circumstances of vagueness.

Elisabeth Rakus-Andersson: *Fuzzy and Rough Techniques in Medical Diagnosis and Medication*,
StudFuzz **212**, 3–30 (2007)
www.springerlink.com 

## 2.2 Fuzzy Sets

If we use the expression "a set" we will interpret it as a given collection of objects that are listed exactly, or that have the same property. Define $A = \{4,5,6,7\}$. The set $A$ contains a determined number of elements and it thus is called a finite set. If we cannot count the number of elements in a set, e.g., $B = \{1,2,3,4,5,6,7,\ldots\}$ we will call $B$ an infinite set.

Let us introduce a function $\mu_C$ as a characteristic function of a crisp set $C$. The crisp set $C$ of universe $X = \{x\}$ is represented by its characteristic function $\mu_C$ as follows.

**Definition 2.1**

The function $\mu_C : X \to \{0,1\}$ is the characteristic function of the set $C$ if and only if for all $x \in X$

$$y = \mu_C(x) = \begin{cases} 1 & \text{for} \quad x \in C, \\ 0 & \text{for} \quad x \notin C. \end{cases} \tag{2.1}$$

**Example 2.1**

Figure 2.1 shows the characteristic function of the crisp set $C = [4, 8]$.

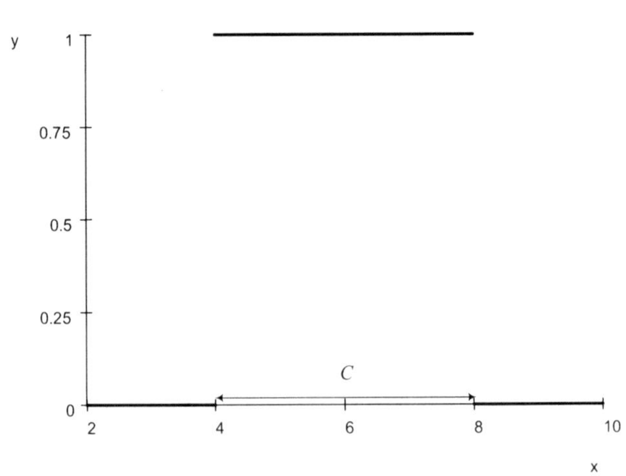


Figure 2.1: The characteristic function of the crisp set $C = [4, 8]$

In *fuzzy set theory* classical sets are called *crisp sets* in order to distinguish them from *fuzzy sets*. Let $C$ be a crisp set defined with the domain named $X$. Then for any element $x \in X$ (the sign "$\in$" denotes that an element $x$ belongs to the set $X$) we have that $x \in C$ or $x \notin C$ if the sign "$\notin$" stands for "does not belong". In fuzzy set theory this property is generalized. Therefore, in fuzzy set $A$, it is not necessary that either $x \in A$ or $x \notin A$ [10, 12, 14, 40, 41, 44, 48, 54, 55, 69, 88, 89, 95].

The generalization is assumed as follows. According to the above statement for any crisp set $C$ it is possible to define a characteristic function $\mu_C : X \to \{0, 1\}$. In fuzzy set theory, the above characteristic function is generalized to *a membership function* that assigns every $x \in X$ a value from the unit interval [0, 1] instead of being assigned from the two-element set $\{0, 1\}$. The set $A$, defined on the basis of a generalized characteristic function, is called a fuzzy set.

**Definition 2.2**

The membership function $\mu_A$ of fuzzy set $A$ is a function defined as $\mu_A : X \to [0, 1]$. Every element $x \in X$ has thus *a membership degree* $y = \mu_A(x) \in [0, 1]$. The fuzzy set $A$ is finally completely determined by the set of pairs

$$A = \{(x, y) = (x, \mu_A(x))\} \ , \ x \in X. \tag{2.2}$$

**Definition 2.3**

The important part of fuzzy set $A$ is *a support* denoted by supp($A$) and defined as a non-fuzzy set (the sign ":" denotes "for which") [40, 88, 95]

$$\mathrm{supp}(A) = \{x \in X : \mu_A(x) > 0\}. \tag{2.3}$$

**Example 2.2**

Suppose that fuzzy set $A$ has the support supp($A$) = $\{x : 0 \le x \le 10\}$, and its membership function is given by

$$y = \mu_A(x) = \begin{cases} \frac{1}{3}x & \text{for} \quad 0 \le x < 3, \\ 1 & \text{for} \quad 3 \le x < 8, \\ -\frac{1}{2}x + 5 & \text{for} \quad 8 \le x \le 10 . \end{cases}$$

By analyzing the last formula we can sketch the membership function of $A$ as a graph placed in Fig. 2.2.

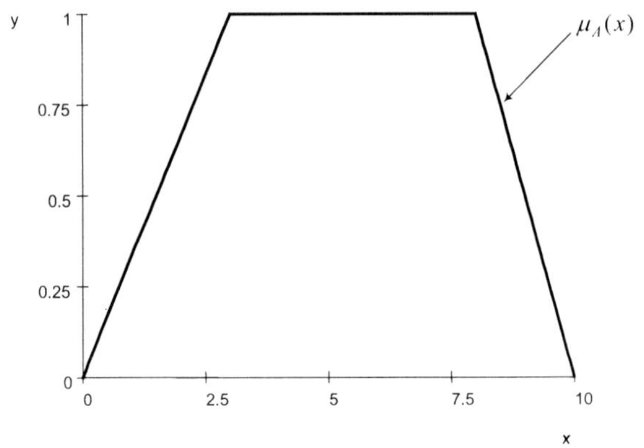


Figure 2.2: Fuzzy set $A = \{(x, \mu_A(x))\}, x \in [0, 10]$

Fuzzy sets are extremely useful when we want to formalize mathematically the descriptions of some uncertain occurrences. How do we define such sets as, for example, "*young*", "*old*" or "*cold*"? We may not decide that the maximal value in the set "*young*" will be 25. The age "26" should be included in "*young*" as well but the association of 26 with "*young*" will be weaker, for instance, 0.9 instead of 1.

**Example 2.3**

Let us state the non-fuzzy finite set "*young*" = {18, 20, 25, 30, 35, 40, 45, 50}, and let us intuitively decide strength of the relationship between the set and each value belonging to its support.

$$\text{"}young\text{"} = \{(18,1),(20,1),(25,0.9),(30,0.7),(35,0.5),(40,0.3),(45,0.1),(50,0)\}$$

that now becomes the fuzzy set that can be listed in another shape as

$$\text{"}young\text{"} = 1/18 + 1/20 + 0.9/25 + 0.7/30 + 0.5/35 + 0.3/40 + 0.1/45 + 0/50 .$$

We explain that the number over the slash constitutes a value of the membership degree of an element $x$. The element $x$ is placed under the slash. The sign "+" links members of the set and has only a symbolic meaning.

If we design the membership function of the continuous set "*young*" as the figure with boundary lines

$$y = \mu_{"young"}(x) = \begin{cases} 1 & \text{for} \quad 0 \le x < 25, \\ -\dfrac{1}{25}x + 2 & \text{for} \quad 25 \le x \le 50, \end{cases}$$

then we will obtain the membership degree of an arbitrary age that belongs to [0, 50] in conformity with a graph displayed in Fig. 2.3.

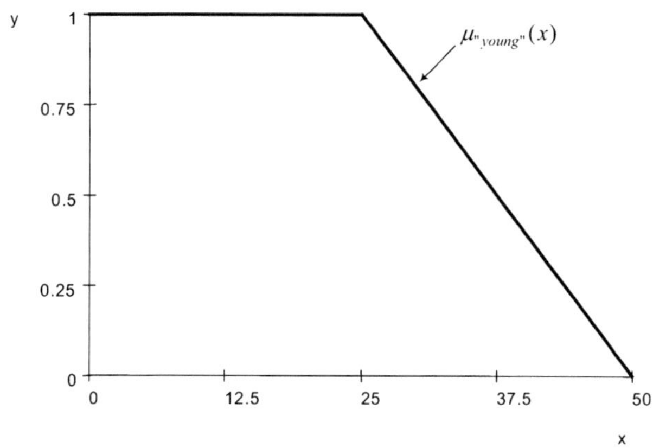


Figure 2.3: The continuous fuzzy set "*young*"

By examining the membership function sketched in the graph we are able to establish the connection between a value of age, e.g., $x = 33$ and the set "*young*" as nearly 0.7. The number indicates the strength of the relationship between the age of 33 and the notion of "*young*".

When the domain $X$ of fuzzy set $A$ is continuous, then the membership function $\mu_A$ will be regarded as a continuous membership function. We will designate $A$ as a symbolic sum

$$A = \sum_{x \in X} \mu_A(x) \Big/ x = \{(x, y) = (x, \mu_A(x))\}, x \in X, \tag{2.4}$$

for which the Σ-sign denotes an infinite enumeration of its elements.

The membership function of a fuzzy set, which has the graph designed as a collection of straight lines linked piece by piece, is the easiest one to apply. However, the split linear function does not yield the only possibility of expressing an association between the set and its elements. We can – as a prognosis of the mentioned relationship – introduce other functions that are continuous and map the support of a fuzzy set onto the interval [0, 1]. As an alternative membership function of the fuzzy set $A$ we demonstrate the $s$-class function $s(x, \alpha, \beta, \gamma)$ with the parameters $\alpha$, $\beta$ and $\gamma$ that are included in the formula [2, 3, 12, 40, 41, 49, 50, 67, 70, 91]

$$y = \mu_A(x) = s(x,\alpha,\beta,\gamma) = \begin{cases} 0 & \text{for } x \le \alpha, \\ 2\left(\dfrac{x-\alpha}{\gamma-\alpha}\right)^2 & \text{for } \alpha < x \le \beta, \\ 1-2\left(\dfrac{x-\gamma}{\gamma-\alpha}\right)^2 & \text{for } \beta < x \le \gamma, \\ 1 & \text{for } x > \gamma, \end{cases} \tag{2.5}$$

where $\beta = \dfrac{\alpha+\gamma}{2}$.

**Example 2.4**

The function $s(x, 25, 37.5, 50)$ is plotted in Fig. 2.4.

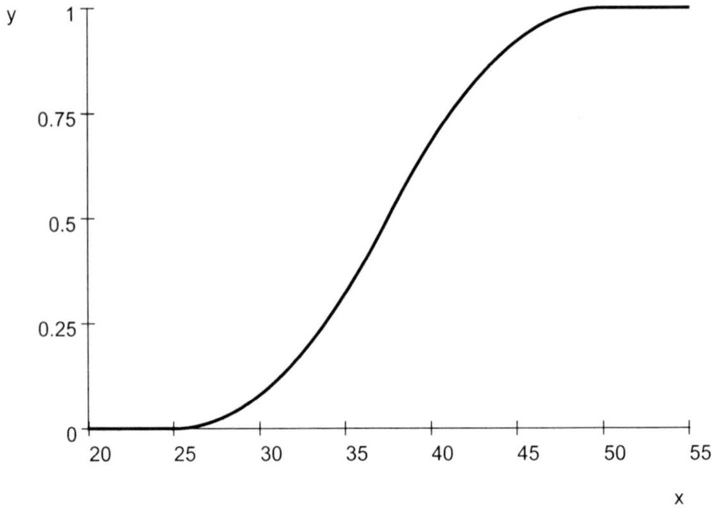


Figure 2.4: The function $s(x, 25, 37.5, 50)$

The $s$-function holds a number of properties that stand out as very advantageous. As a continuous polynomial of the second degree the $s$-function can assist further analytical operations, such as differentiation or integration without making them very complicated. It is also evident from the formula (2.5) that the range of $s$ covers the interval [0, 1] that is a desirable feature of the membership function.

**Example 2.5**

By proposing the membership function of the set "*young*" as a formula $\mu_{\text{"young"}}(x) = 1 - s(x, 25, 37.5, 50)$ we create another relationship between the concept of "*young*" and its elements when comparing to Ex. 2.3. Figure 2.5 interprets the alternative set "*young*".

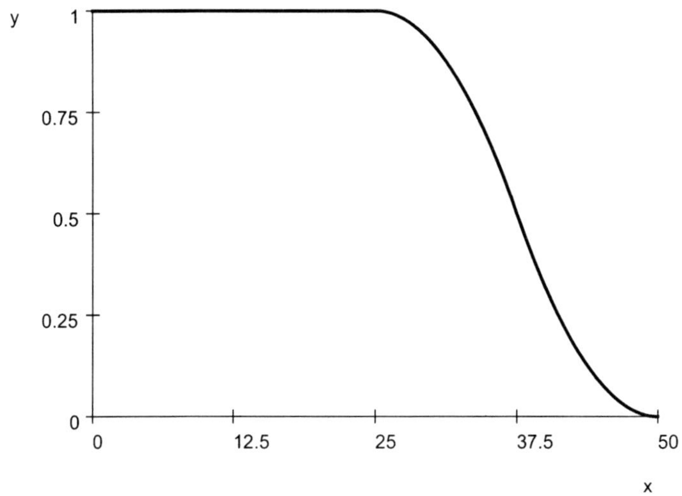


Figure 2.5: The membership function of the set "*young*" as the $s$-class function

The same value of age can be a member of many sets with different membership degrees. Let us introduce three sets named "*young*", "*middle-aged*" and "*old*". To suggest a membership function of the set "*middle-aged*" we test a function of the $\pi$-class constructed as

$$y = \pi(x, \alpha, \beta) = \begin{cases} s\left(x, \beta - \alpha, \beta - \dfrac{\alpha}{2}, \beta\right) & \text{for} \quad x \le \beta, \\ 1 - s\left(x, \beta, \beta + \dfrac{\alpha}{2}, \beta + \alpha\right) & \text{for} \quad x > \beta. \end{cases} \tag{2.6}$$

**Example 2.6**

When we decide $\alpha = 20$ and $\beta = 45$, we will accommodate (2.6) to the formula

$$y = \pi(x,20,45) = \begin{cases} s(x,25,35,45) & \text{for} \quad x \leq 45, \\ 1 - s(x,45,55,65) & \text{for} \quad x > 45. \end{cases}$$

The graph of $\pi(x, 20, 45)$ is drawn in Fig. 2.6.

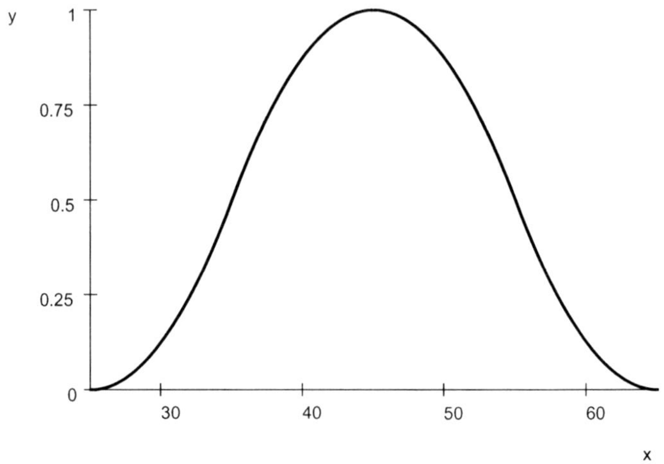


Figure 2.6: The function $\pi(x, 20, 45)$

By constructing three fuzzy sets with supports that overlap each other we demonstrate again the idea of imprecision in the following task.

**Example 2.7**

Three fuzzy sets of the universe $X = [0, 100]$, made for different groups of age, are now put forward as "*young*" with $y = \mu_{\text{"young"}}(x) = 1 - s(x, 25, 37.5, 50)$, "*middle-aged*" with $y = \mu_{\text{"middle-aged"}}(x) = \pi(x, 20, 45)$ and, finally, "*old*" characterized by the membership function $y = \mu_{\text{"old"}}(x) = s(x, 40, 52.5, 65)$. The sets have no sharp borders; on the contrary, some non-empty intersections of all supports are built in the sets' domains. Figure 2.7 visually explains the concept of vagueness even better since it helps us to understand the effects of fuzziness when studying the sets that are not disjoint in spite of the different classifiers of age.

We compute that $x = 42$ belongs to "*young*" with the membership degree equal 0.2048 because of $y = 1 - s(42, 25, 37.5, 50) = 1 - \left(1 - 2\left(\dfrac{42-50}{50-25}\right)^2\right), 42 \in (37.5, 50]$.

The connection between $x = 42$ and "*middle-aged*" is evaluated as 0.955 in relation to $y(42) = s(42, 25, 35, 45)$. The value of $x = 42$ is not a member of the set "*old*".

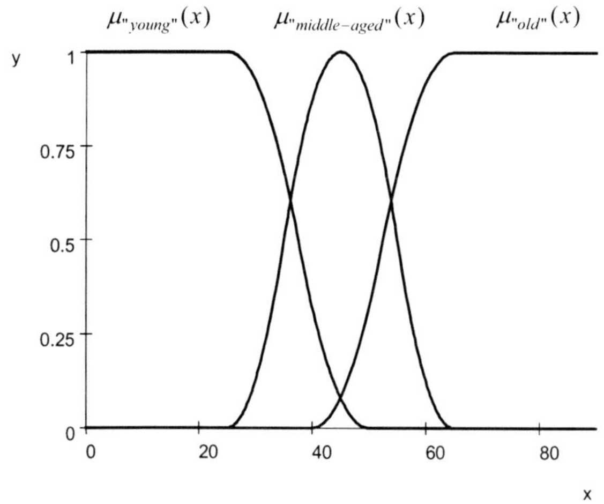


Figure 2.7: The fuzzy sets "*young*", "*middle-aged*" and "*old*" in $X = [0, 100]$

Measurable, medical parameters can be interpreted as fuzzy sets to prepare data to models described in the next parts of this work. Clinical symptoms involved in mathematical decision patterns will be represented by values of membership degrees. The degrees, as numbers, express the intensities of symptom presence or symptom importance without engaging in complicated verbal descriptions. The possibility of computing with words, which are replaced by real numbers assigned to them, facilitates the communication among researchers who represent different scientific fields.

**Example 2.8**

The existence of fuzzy sets enables an introduction of medical models that operate with clinical symptoms constituting the basis for a decision. To evaluate the importance of increasing body temperature via a corresponding membership degree, we propose adopting the fuzzy set "*body temperature*" with a membership function expanded by

$$y = \mu_{\text{"body temperature"}}(x) = \begin{cases} 1 - s(x, 35°, 35.8°, 36.6°) & \text{for} \quad 35° \le x \le 36.6°, \\ s(x, 36.6°, 39.3°, 42°) & \text{for} \quad 36.6° < x \le 42°. \end{cases}$$

The membership function of the set "*body temperature*" is sketched in Fig. 2.8. The values of membership degrees provide us with an estimation of the temperature importance for states in which body temperature is too high or too low in comparison to its normal value.

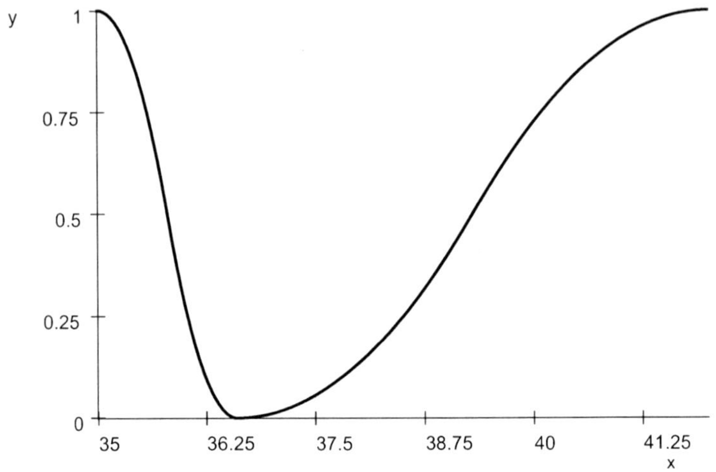


Figure 2.8: The membership function of the set "*body temperature*"

## 2.3 Basic Operations on Fuzzy Sets

The definition of a fuzzy set that differs from the concept of a crisp set has entailed new approaches to the operations on fuzzy sets. In order to connect two fuzzy sets let us study their union and intersection.

At first, we recall the classical operation of the union performed on two non-fuzzy sets.

**Definition 2.4**

The union of two crisp sets $A = \{x : x \in A\}$ and $B = \{x : x \in B\}$, $A, B \subset X = \{\mathrm{x}\}$ (denoted by "$\cup$") is a set $A \cup B = \{x : x \in A \text{ or } x \in B\}$. We remember that the sign ":" is read as "for which".

In practice, the set $A \cup B$ is a collection of all elements that belong to either $A$ or $B$ provided that identical elements are counted only once.

**Example 2.9**

For $A = [2, 6]$ and $B = [4, 9]$ the union is determined as $A \cup B = [2, 9]$.

A union of two fuzzy sets should also be a fuzzy set. By accepting the operation of the classical union for the supports of fuzzy sets, we establish a common support of the union of fuzzy sets while the connective union operation for membership degrees can be suggested in the following definition.

**Definition 2.5**

Let $A = \{(x, \mu_A(x))\}$ and $B = \{(x, \mu_B(x))\}$, $x \in X$, denote two fuzzy sets. The union of $A$ and $B$ is a fuzzy set $A \cup B = \{(x, \mu_{A \cup B}(x))\}$, $x \in (\text{supp}(A) \cup \text{supp}(B))$, for which the membership function is given by [12, 40, 88, 95]

$$\mu_{A \cup B}(x) = \max_{x \in (\text{supp}(A) \cup \text{supp}(B))} (\mu_A(x), \mu_B(x)). \tag{2.7}$$

**Example 2.10**

If $A$ has $\text{supp}(A) = [2, 6]$ and $\mu_A(x) = 1 - s(x, 2, 4, 6)$, while $B$ is fixed precisely by $\text{supp}(B) = [4, 9]$ and $\mu_B(x) = s(x, 4, 6.5, 9)$, then the union of $A$ and $B$ will consist of $\text{supp}(A \cup B) = [2, 9]$ and $\mu_{A \cup B}(x) = \max(1 - s(x, 2, 4, 6),\ s(x, 4, 6.5, 9))$ for every $x \in [2, 9]$ in accordance with a dotted curve placed in Fig. 2.9.

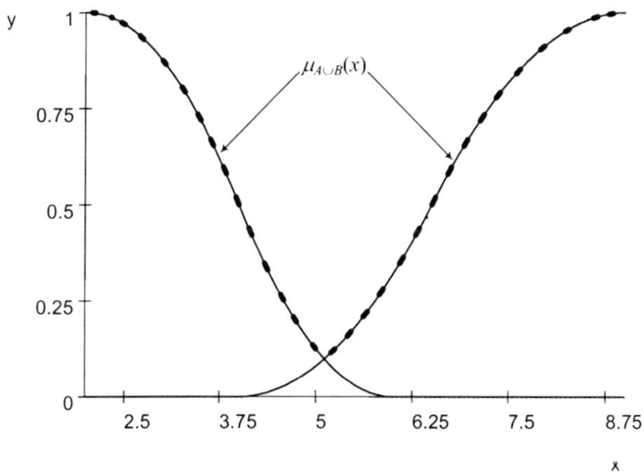


Figure 2.9: The union of fuzzy sets $A$ and $B$ from Ex. 2.10

In order to estimate the membership degree of, e.g., $x = 4.5$ in the union $A \cup B$ we will follow the expression $\mu_{A \cup B}(4.5) = \max(1 - s(4.5, 2, 4, 6), s(4.5, 4, 6.5, 9))$

$$= \max\left\{1 - \left[1 - 2\left(\frac{4.5-6}{4}\right)^2\right], 2\left(\frac{4.5-4}{5}\right)^2\right\} = \max(0.28125, 0.02) = 0.28125.$$

The replacement of the operation "max" in the membership function of the union of the two fuzzy sets $A$ and $B$ by the dual operation "min", generates an intersection of $A$ and $B$. We state that a support of the intersection between $A$ and $B$ is composed of these elements that take place in the union of the sets' supports. Since some elements of the intersection get the membership degrees equal to zero, then we should reduce the common support to its essential part in which is $\mu_{A\cap B}(x) > 0$.

**Definition 2.6**

For $A = \{(x, \mu_A(x))\}$ and $B = \{(x, \mu_B(x))\}$, $x \in X$, that are two fuzzy sets, the intersection of $A$ and $B$, marked by "$\cap$", is a fuzzy set $A \cap B = \{(x, \mu_{A\cap B}(x))\}$ for all $x \in (\mathrm{supp}(A) \cup \mathrm{supp}(B))$. Its membership function is shaped by [12, 40, 88, 95]

$$\mu_{A\cap B}(x) = \min_{x\in(\mathrm{supp}(A)\cup\mathrm{supp}(B))} (\mu_A(x), \mu_B(x)). \tag{2.8}$$

**Example 2.11**

For the sets $A$ and $B$ from Ex. 2.10 the membership function of the intersection is indicated by the dotted line drawn in Fig. 2.10.

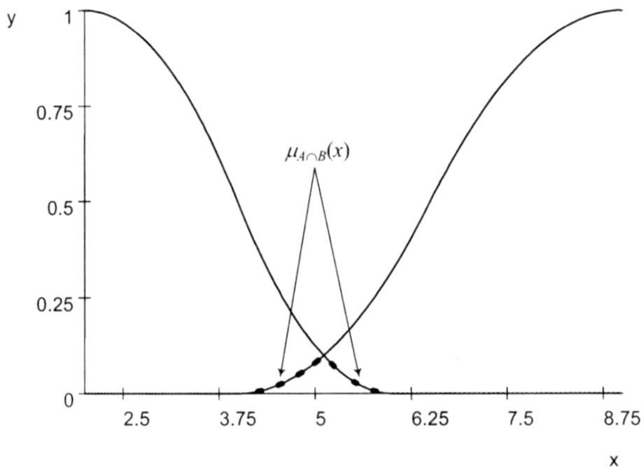


Figure 2.10: The intersection of $A$ and $B$ from Ex. 2.10

There also exists the complement of fuzzy set $A$ introduced by the following definition [12, 40, 88, 95].

**Definition 2.7**

Let $A = \{(x, \mu_A(x))\}$, $x \in X$. The complement of $A$, denoted $A^`$, is a fuzzy set with the membership function $\mu_{A^`}$ given by the formula

$$\mu_{A'}(x) = 1 - \mu_A(x), \text{ for } x \in X. \tag{2.9}$$

**Example 2.12**

Suppose that $B$ – the fuzzy set examined in Ex. 2.10 – is determined by supp($B$) = [4, 9] and $\mu_B(x) = s(x, 4, 6.5, 9)$. We thus establish a membership function of the complement $B$` as the curve presented by Fig. 2.11 for these $x$ that belong to supp($B$).

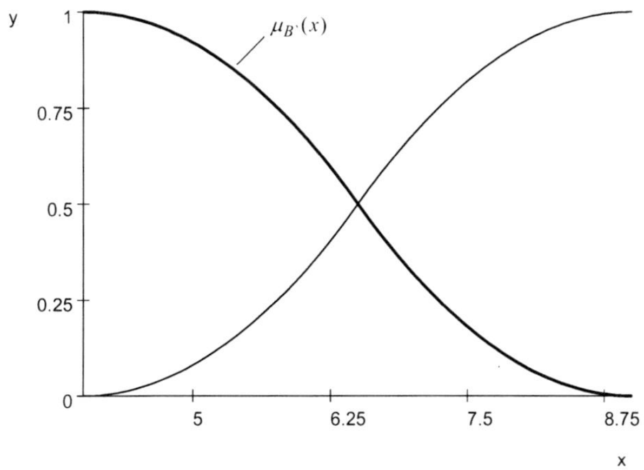


Figure 2.11: The complement of the set $B$ from Ex. 2.10

Let us discuss another example that inserts a simple and practical aspect of the union and the intersection of two fuzzy sets.

**Example 2.13**

We consider two fuzzy sets "*young*" and "*experienced*" in the space of ages $X$ = [0, 100]. The set "*young*" is still determined by the membership function

$$\mu_{\text{"}young\text{"}}(x) = \begin{cases} 1 & \text{for} \quad 0 \le x < 25, \\ -\dfrac{1}{25}x + 2 & \text{for} \quad 25 \le x < 50, \\ 0 & \text{for} \quad 50 \le x \le 100, \end{cases}$$

in accordance with Ex. 2.3. The rule "*more experienced with growing age*" suggests a creation of the set "*experienced*" as a fuzzy set related to the membership function

$$\mu_{\text{"experienced"}}(x) = \begin{cases} 0 & \text{for} \quad 0 \le x < 15, \\ \frac{1}{45}x - \frac{1}{3} & \text{for} \quad 15 \le x < 60, \\ 1 & \text{for} \quad 60 \le x \le 100. \end{cases}$$

The adaptation of (2.7) to a union of the sets "*young*" and "*experienced*" causes the existence of a fuzzy set "*young or experienced*" with the membership function

$$\mu_{\text{"young or experienced"}}(x) = \begin{cases} 1 & \text{for} \quad 0 \le x < 25, \\ -\frac{1}{25}x + 2 & \text{for} \quad 25 \le x < 37.63, \\ \frac{1}{45}x - \frac{1}{3} & \text{for} \quad 37.63 \le x < 60, \\ 1 & \text{for} \quad 60 \le x \le 100, \end{cases}$$

that is depicted in Fig. 2.12.

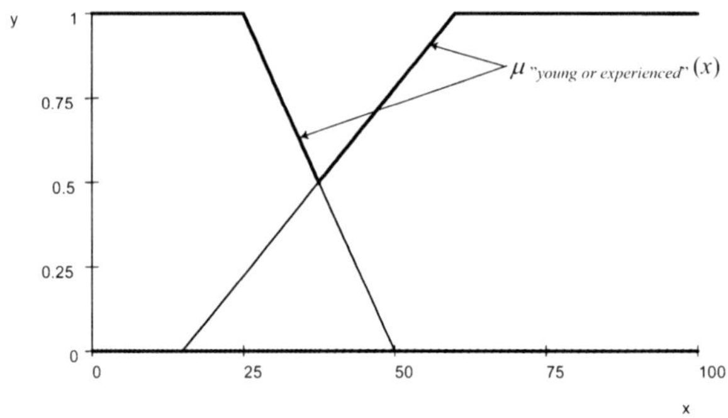


Figure 2.12: The membership function of the set "*young or experienced*"

Equation (2.8) is a tool of deciding an intersection "*young and experienced*" of the sets "*young*" and "*experienced*". This intersection, being a fuzzy set, is modelled by the function

$$\mu_{\text{"young and experienced"}}(x) = \begin{cases} 0 & \text{for} \quad 0 \le x < 15, \\ \frac{1}{45}x - \frac{1}{3} & \text{for} \quad 15 \le x < 37.63, \\ -\frac{1}{25}x + 2 & \text{for} \quad 37.63 \le x < 50, \\ 0 & \text{for} \quad 50 \le x \le 100. \end{cases}$$

Figure 2.13 proposes the graph of "*young and experienced*".

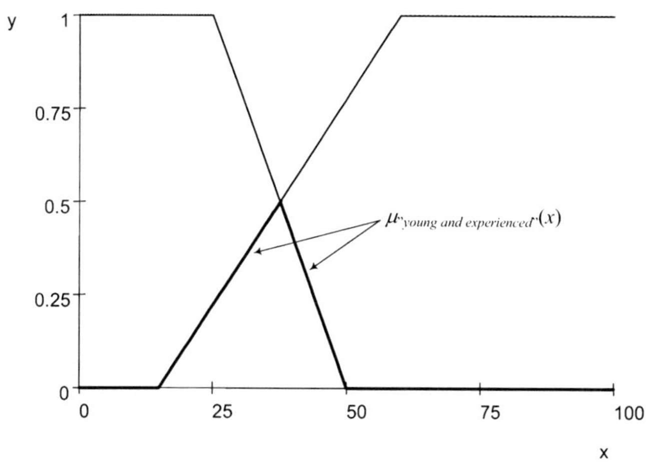


Figure 2.13: The membership function of the set "*young and experienced*"

It is easy to verify that the membership function of the intersection operation (2.8) then rewritten as

$$\mu_{A \cap B}(x) = \min_{x \in X}(\mu_A(x), \mu_B(x)) = t(\mu_A(x), \mu_B(x)) \tag{2.10}$$

is a function from [0, 1] × [0, 1] into [0, 1]. The sign "×", used symbolically as a notion of the Cartesian product, informs us that we should take a pair of two numbers from [0, 1] to map this pair of quantities in another number belonging to the interval [0, 1] as well. The minimum function satisfies some pre-defined properties. If other functions behave themselves like the minimum, then we should generate for them a class of functions named *t*-norms. The *t*-norms have the following features

$$\begin{aligned}
&1.\ t(0,0)=0;\ t(\mu_A(x),1)=t(1,\mu_A(x))=\mu_A(x), x\in X,\\
&2.\ t(\mu_A(x),\mu_B(x))\le t(\mu_C(x),\mu_D(x)) \text{ if } \mu_A(x)\le\mu_C(x) \text{ and } \mu_{\text{\textit{l}}}\\
&3.\ t(\mu_A(x),\mu_B(x))=t(\mu_B(x),\mu_A(x)),\\
&4.\ t(\mu_A(x),t(\mu_B(x),\mu_C(x)))=t(t(\mu_A(x),\mu_B(x)),\mu_C(x)).
\end{aligned} \tag{2.11}$$

For minimum the first condition is fulfilled because $t(0, 0) = \min(0, 0) = 0$ and $t(\mu_A(x), 1) = \min(\mu_A(x), 1) = \mu_A(\mathrm{x})$.

The minimum operator is a *t-norm* [12, 41, 44, 95]. If we define any function $t(a, b) = c$ for $a, b, c \in [0, 1]$, $t : [0,1] \times [0,1] \rightarrow [0,1]$, due to conditions 1-4 in (2.11) we will form another intersection operation for two fuzzy sets, e.g., the bounded product, the algebraic product, the Einstein product, the Yager product and the like [44, 95]. To watch the difference between the minimum norm, called also the largest norm, and the bounded norm defined as

$$t(\mu_A(x),\mu_B(x)) = \max_{x\in X}(\mu_A(x)+\mu_B(x)-1,0) \tag{2.12}$$

we compare a value of the $t$-minimum norm for a pair, e.g., (0.8, 0,5) equal to min(0.8, 0.5) = 0.5 to the $t$-bounded norm value calculated as max(0.8 + 0.5 – 1, 0) = 0.3.

The membership function (2.7) of the union of two fuzzy sets that is interpreted as the function

$$\mu_{A\cup B}(x) = \max_{x\in X}(\mu_A(x),\mu_B(x)) = s(\mu_A(x),\mu_B(x)), \tag{2.13}$$

also is a mapping from $[0,1] \times [0,1]$ into $[0,1]$ with the following properties

$$\begin{aligned}
&1.\ s(1,1)=1;\ s(\mu_A(x),0)=s(0,\mu_A(x))=\mu_A(x),\ x\in X,\\
&2.\ s(\mu_A(x),\mu_B(x))\le s(\mu_C(x),\mu_D(x))\\
&\quad \text{if } \mu_A(x)\le\mu_C(x) \text{ and } \mu_B(x)\le\mu_D(x),\\
&3.\ s(\mu_A(x),\mu_B(x))=s(\mu_B(x),\mu_A(x)),\\
&4.\ s(\mu_A(x),s(\mu_B(x),\mu_C(x)))=s(s(\mu_A(x),\mu_B(x)),\mu_C(x)).
\end{aligned} \tag{2.14}$$

When checking for the maximum, the reliability of the first condition from (2.14), we state that $s(1, 1) = \max(1, 1) = 1$ and $s(\mu_A(x), 0) = \max(\mu_A(x), 0) = \mu_A(x)$.

The function $s(a, b) = c$, $a, b, c \in [0, 1]$, is called an *s-norm* (coincidentally the same notion like the $s$-function $s(x, \alpha, \beta, \gamma)$). If we propose another definition satisfying the features 1-4 in (2.14) we will create a class of union operations on fuzzy sets.

The operations concatenating two fuzzy sets will constitute an important basis for solutions to medical projects.

## 2.4 Linguistic Variables

The conception of a variable in classical mathematics makes us think of joining a number to a name of a certain symbol, usually denoted by the letters $x$, $y$, $z$ and the like. Nobody doubts that the classical variable takes values associated with it for a hundred percent certainty. In fuzzy set theory we join values to the name of a variable even if the values reveal a weaker relationship with the variable than a "sure connection".

The assigned values to a variable need not be numbers. It is possible to use some words or some structures to express a connection between the name of the variable and its range if the connection is imprecise and cannot be described exactly.

If we think about the idea of a variable then we can imagine constructing an equation

$$x = a \tag{2.15}$$

that assigns a value of $a$ to the name $x$.

Generally, let us accept the name of the variable as $X$ and let us recognize $A$ as a set of all values taken by $X$. The set $A$ is called the range of $X$. If we further restrict the values of the range $A$ by imposing a constraint $R(X) \subseteq A$ on the values of $X$, it will mean that $X$ takes only the values that belong to $R(X)$. A new equation that assigns the value of $a$ to $X$ is derived as

$$x = a,\ a \in R(X)\,. \tag{2.16}$$

Suppose that the constraint $R(X)$ is a fuzzy set. The variable $X$, which takes its values in the range $A$ and possesses the fuzzy constraint $R(X)$, is now renamed as *a fuzzy variable* [28, 40, 90, 95]. The values assigned to $X$ are the elements of a fuzzy set (a fuzzy constraint) and thus they are equipped with a corresponding membership degree.

By using the equation (2.16) we make the next trial of associating the variable $X$ and its values provided that (2.16) is supplemented by a so-called *compatibility degree* $c(a) \in [0, 1]$. The mentioned equation (2.16) is now rewritten in the form of

$$x = a,\ c(a) = \mu_{R(X)}(a),\ a \in \text{supp}(R(x)),\ c(a) \in [0,1]\,. \tag{2.17}$$

The compatibility degree $c(a)$ is computed for the value of $a$ by adopting a formula of the membership function defined for $R(X)$.

**Example 2.14**

Let us examine the relation between a certain diagnosis $D$ and one of clinical symptoms typical of $D$ that is named $S$. The relationship between $S$ and $D$ can illustrate a concept of the fuzzy variable. We pose a question referring to the frequency of the symptom present in the selected diagnosis. We expect – as an answer – such a frequency description like, e.g., "*often*", "*seldom*", "*never*", "*almost always*" and other formulations related to intensity of the symptom present. We use words as the answers but we wish to convert them into numbers that intend to represent the linguistic structures in future computations.

Suppose that a basic reference to set $A = \{0, 1, 2, \ldots, 100\}$ includes one hundred patients. We determine the name of a fuzzy variable $X$ as "*often*". Let a fuzzy set $R$("*often*") be the fuzzy constraint laid on the set $A$ by the variable $X$. The membership function of $R$("*often*") is given by the formula

$$\mu_{R(\text{"often"})}(a) = s(a,50,60,70),$$

that is interpreted in the explicit form, in accordance with (2.5), as

$$y = \mu_{R(\text{"often"})}(a) = s(a,50,60,70) = \begin{cases} 0 & \text{for} \quad a \le 50, \\ 2\left(\dfrac{a-50}{70-50}\right)^2 & \text{for} \quad \text{for } 50 < a \le 60, \\ 1-2\left(\dfrac{a-70}{70-50}\right)^2 & \text{for} \quad 60 < a \le 70, \\ 1 & \text{for} \quad a > 70. \end{cases}$$

The appearance of a curve plotted in Fig. 2.14 is an instance of influence of the constraint $R$("*often*") on the range of the reference set $A$. It is no doubt that a status of the variable name gives rise to the selection of the parameters $\alpha$, $\beta$ and $\gamma$ placed in the membership function of $R$("*often*").

Figure 2.14: The constraint $R$("*often*") over the reference set $A = [0, 100]$

In the equation "*often*" = 40, $c(40) = 0$, the compatibility between the value of 40 and the frequency notion "*often*" is equal to zero in the space of one hundred patients. If "*often*" = 58 then $c(58) = 2\left(\dfrac{58-50}{70-50}\right)^2 = 0.32$. The grade indicates that the strength of the connection between the name "*often*" and a sample of fifty-eight patients in comparison with one hundred patients is appreciated as 0.32. Another equation – "*often*" = 72, $c(72) = 1$ – confirms the total compatibility between the name of the variable "*often*" and its value 72.

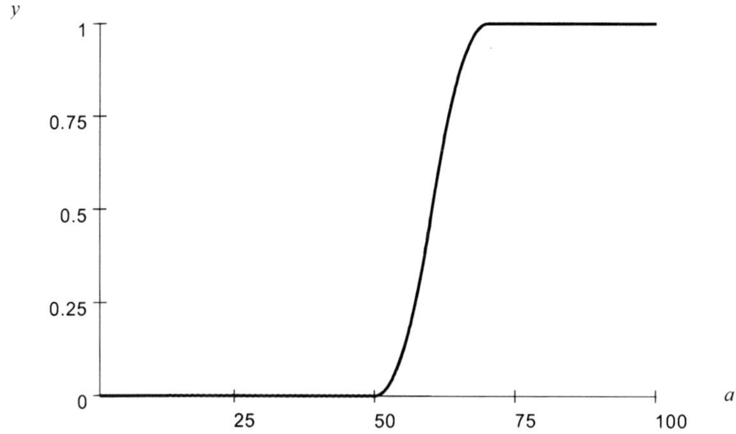


Figure 2.14: The constraint $R$("*often*") over the reference set $A = [0, 100]$

The introduction of the fuzzy variable "*often*" allows us to replace the word *often* by the set of numbers that are associated with this linguistic item. However, we realize that we should operate with many more words or structures to describe a certain occurrence like, e.g., *intensity of presence* introduced in Ex. 2.14. In other words, we want to have at our disposal a full list of words, and moreover, we would like to be able to express every word in the form of a number set in the common space. This idea contributes to the evolution of a variable range by giving access as verbal expressions as its members. A *linguistic variable* that offers commonly used words as its range characters is interpreted as such.

The linguistic variable is a variable taking values expressed by words. These are names of fuzzy variables defined in a space such as $A = \{0, 1, 2, \ldots, 100\}$. Let us denote the linguistic variable by $L$ and a set of its terms by $T = \{T_1, T_2, \ldots, T_n\}$, where each $T_i$, $i = 1, 2, \ldots, n$, is the name of a fuzzy variable restricted by a fuzzy constraint $R(T_i)$ definable in the space $A$. An equation

$$L = T_i, i = 1, \ldots, n \tag{2.18}$$

that links a "value" $T_i$ to the linguistic variable $L$, reveals a relation between a general name of the variable and one of its semantic terms.

**Example 2.15**

Suppose that we are able to upgrade the frequency of a symptom in the associated diagnosis by employing average verbal expressions that emphasize the importance of symptom presence. We can thus utilize a list of words to make a conversation with a cooperating physician much more comfortable. We should realize that the physician must experience some difficulties in telling us his opinion as a strict mathematical number that describes the grade of symptom presence. Let us decide a content $T$ of the list "*presence of symptom S in diagnosis D*" as $T = \{T_1 =$ "*never*", $T_2 =$ "*almost never*", $T_3 =$ "*very seldom*", $T_4 =$ "*seldom*", $T_5 =$ "*moderately*", $T_6 =$ "*often*", $T_7 =$ "*very often*", $T_8 =$ "*almost always*", $T_9 =$ "*always*"$\}$. Each of the terms from the list constitutes the name of a fuzzy variable placed in the reference set $A = \{0, 1, 2, \ldots, 100\}$. In order to characterize the intervals in the set of one hundred patients that are typical of the names from the list, the following restrictions are put forward by their membership functions [2, 3, 56]

$$\mu_{R(T_1=\text{"never"})}(a) = 1 - s(a,0,5,10),$$

$$\mu_{R(T_2=\text{"almost never"})}(a) = 1 - s(a,6,10,14),$$

$$\mu_{R(T_3=\text{"very seldom"})}(a) = 1 - s(a,15,20,25),$$

$$\mu_{R(T_4=\text{"seldom"})}(a) = 1 - s(a,30,40,50),$$

$$\mu_{R(T_5=\text{"moderately"})}(a) = \pi(a,20,50),$$

$$\mu_{R(T_6=\text{"often"})}(a) = s(a,50,60,70),$$

$$\mu_{R(T_7=\text{"very often"})}(a) = s(a,75,80,85),$$

$$\mu_{R(T_8=\text{"almost always"})}(a) = s(a,86,90,94),$$

$$\mu_{R(T_9=\text{"always"})}(a) = s(a,90,95,100).$$

Figure 2.15 gives an impression of dividing space $A$ into subintervals that selects the terms assigned to the linguistic variable "*presence of symptom S in diagnosis D*". It is remarkable to notice that the intervals build non-disjointed intersections. The occurrence of overlapping the supports of fuzzy sets emphasizes fuzzy performance of sets once again.

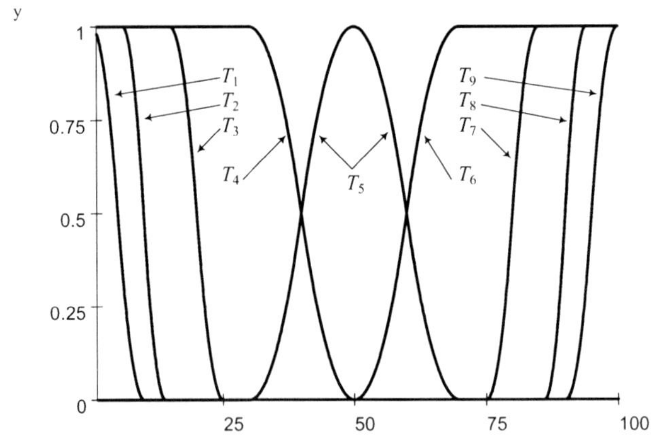


Figure 2.15: The fuzzy constraints of terms representing "*presence of S in D*"

The boundary values of fuzzy constraints from Fig. 2.15 have been decided in compliance with the physician's advice. In one of the next chapters we intend to introduce formal, mathematical evidence that explains how to construct fuzzy restrictions for terms belonging to the list of a linguistic variable. The concept of atomic words and hedges will be involved in the evidence as conclusive factors of the solutions.

An equation, in which a term is attributed to the variable name, determines the relationship between the linguistic variable, e.g., "*presence of symptom S in diagnosis D*" and one of its terms such as "*almost never*". In this way we can state the connection

$$\text{"}\textit{presence of symptom } S \textit{ in diagnosis } D\text{"} = \text{"}\textit{almost never}\text{"} .$$

The notions of fuzzy variables and linguistic variables constitute very important tools in medical models that are discussed in the next chapters. The linguistic variable makes it possible to convert words or other verbal structures into numbers, and this possibility then opens up an understandable dialogue between physicians and mathematicians working together.

## 2.5 Fuzzy Relations

Fuzzy relations join two-non fuzzy sets in the common set of pairs on condition that each pair has the membership degree assigned.

To understand better the idea of a fuzzy relation let us first study the basic definition of a Cartesian product of two non-fuzzy sets.

**Definition 2.8**

Let $X = \{x_1, x_2, \ldots, x_m\}$ and $Y = \{y_1, y_2, \ldots, y_n\}$ be two finite sets. The Cartesian product of $X$ and $Y$, denoted by $X \times Y$, is a set of ordered pairs $(x_i, y_j)$, $i = 1, 2, \ldots, m$, $j = 1, 2, \ldots, n$, for $x_i \in X$ and $y_j \in Y$.

**Example 2.16**

If $X = \{1, 2, 3\}$ and $Y = \{a, b\}$ then $X \times Y = \{(1, a), (1, b), (2, a), (2, b), (3, a), (3, b)\}$.

If each pair $(x_i, y_j)$ included in $X \times Y$ is equipped with a membership degree then the Cartesian product that is mapped in the interval [0, 1] by a membership function, will be called a fuzzy relation. Formally, let us introduce the fuzzy relation $\widetilde{R}$ in the following way [12, 40, 88, 95].

**Definition 2.9**

Let $X = \{x_1, x_2, \ldots, x_m\}$ and $Y = \{y_1, y_2, \ldots, y_n\}$ be two finite sets; then

$$\widetilde{R} = \{((x_i, y_j), \mu_{\widetilde{R}}(x_i, y_j))\}, (x_i, y_j) \in X \times Y, \mu_{\widetilde{R}} : X \times Y \to [0,1] \tag{2.19}$$

for $i = 1, 2, \ldots, m, j = 1, 2, \ldots, n$.

Fuzzy relations are often presented in the form of two-dimensional tables. The rows of such a table are all marked by $x$ while the columns are all indicated by $y$. An entry of the table corresponds to this membership degree of the pair $(x, y)$ that belongs to the intersection of row $x$ and column $y$.

An $m \times n$ table-matrix constitutes a comfortable way of entering the fuzzy relation $\widetilde{R}$ that presents a format suggested below

$$\widetilde{R} = \begin{array}{c} \\ x_1 \\ x_2 \\ \vdots \\ x_m \end{array} \begin{array}{c} \begin{array}{cccc} y_1 & y_2 & \cdots & y_n \end{array} \\ \begin{bmatrix} \mu_{\widetilde{R}}(x_1, y_1) & \mu_{\widetilde{R}}(x_1, y_2) & \cdots & \mu_{\widetilde{R}}(x_1, y_n) \\ \mu_{\widetilde{R}}(x_2, y_1) & \mu_{\widetilde{R}}(x_2, y_2) & \cdots & \mu_{\widetilde{R}}(x_2, y_n) \\ \vdots & \vdots & \ddots & \vdots \\ \mu_{\widetilde{R}}(x_m, y_1) & \mu_{\widetilde{R}}(x_m, y_2) & \cdots & \mu_{\widetilde{R}}(x_m, y_n) \end{bmatrix} \end{array}. \tag{2.20}$$

**Example 2.17**

Let $X$ = "*body height*" = [160, 190] and $Y$ = "*body weight*" = [60, 90] be two sets containing the measurements of two parameters $x$ = "*height*" and $y$ = "*weight*" that are characteristic of the man's silhouette. We design a relation "*a strong and proportional construction of the man's body*"$(x, y) = \widetilde{R}(x, y)$, in which the membership degree values of the pairs computed in accordance with the function [28]

$$z = \mu_{\text{"a strong and proportional construction of the man's body"}}(x, y)$$

$$= \mu_{\widetilde{R}}(x, y) = \begin{cases} 0 & \text{for } x < 160,\ y < 60, \\ \dfrac{x - 160}{60} + \dfrac{y - 60}{60} & \text{for } 160 \le x \le 190,\ 60 \le y \le 90, \\ 1 & \text{for } x > 190,\ y > 90, \end{cases}$$

confirm a grade of adaptation of the physical features to the definition of the relation. For instance, the pair (170, 65) has $\mu_{\tilde{R}}(170,65) = \dfrac{170-160}{60} + \dfrac{65-60}{60} =$ 0.25, while another pair (182, 89) shows the compatibility degree with the definition of the relation estimated as equal to $\mu_{\tilde{R}}(182,89) = \dfrac{182-160}{60} + \dfrac{89-60}{60} =$ 0.85.

The general dependence of the membership degrees $\mu_{\tilde{R}}(x,y)$ on the growth of both biological parameters can be observed in Fig. 2.16.

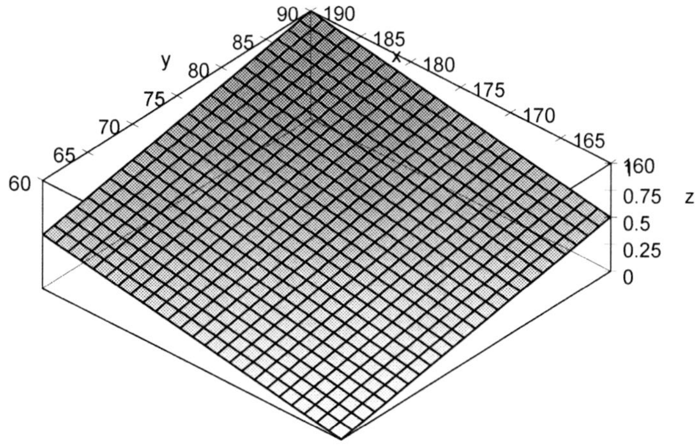


Figure 2.16: "*A strong and proportional construction of the man's body*"

Fuzzy relations can be combined with each other by the operation of "composition". In order to understand better the aggregation of two fuzzy relations, let us first recall the definition of a matrix multiplication for two matrices (dot product).

**Definition 2.10**

If $R = (r_{ij})_{i=1,\ldots,m,\, j=1,\ldots,n}$ and $Q = (q_{jk})_{j=1,\ldots,n,\, k=1,\ldots,p}$ then $S = R \quad Q$ is a product matrix with elements $s_{ik} = \sum_{j=1}^{n} r_{ij} \cdot q_{jk}$, $i = 1, \ldots, m$, $k = 1, \ldots, p$. The number of columns in $R$ must be the same as the row number in $Q$.

The matrices $R$ and $Q$ in table forms are used to clarify the multiplication. Let

$$R=\begin{bmatrix} r_{11} & \cdots & r_{1n} \\ \vdots & \ddots & \vdots \\ r_{m1} & \cdots & r_{mn} \end{bmatrix} \text{ and } Q=\begin{bmatrix} q_{11} & \cdots & q_{1p} \\ \vdots & \ddots & \vdots \\ q_{n1} & \cdots & q_{np} \end{bmatrix}. \text{ Hence, } S=\begin{bmatrix} s_{11} & \cdots & s_{1p} \\ \vdots & \ddots & \vdots \\ s_{m1} & \cdots & s_{mp} \end{bmatrix}$$

$$=\begin{bmatrix} r_{11}\cdot q_{11}+\cdots+r_{1n}\cdot q_{n1} & \cdots & r_{11}\cdot q_{1p}+\cdots+r_{1n}\cdot q_{np} \\ \vdots & \ddots & \vdots \\ r_{m1}\cdot q_{11}+\cdots+r_{mn}\cdot q_{n1} & \cdots & r_{m1}\cdot q_{1p}+\cdots+r_{mn}\cdot q_{np} \end{bmatrix}.$$

**Example 2.18**

We design two matrices $R_{2\times 3}$ and $Q_{3\times 2}$.

Let us multiply the matrices $R=\begin{bmatrix} 2 & 1 & 5 \\ 3 & 6 & 2 \end{bmatrix}$ and $Q=\begin{bmatrix} 4 & 2 \\ 2 & 3 \\ 5 & 7 \end{bmatrix}$.

The product matrix $S$ is obtained in conformity with Def. 2.10 as the matrix

$$S=\begin{bmatrix} 2\cdot 4+1\cdot 2+5\cdot 5 & 2\cdot 2+1\cdot 3+5\cdot 7 \\ 3\cdot 4+6\cdot 2+2\cdot 5 & 3\cdot 2+6\cdot 3+2\cdot 7 \end{bmatrix}=\begin{bmatrix} 35 & 42 \\ 34 & 38 \end{bmatrix}.$$

By returning to fuzzy relations, filled with membership degrees, we will treat the operation of "product" as "composition". To find some adequate operations that replace the external sum and the internal multiplication in the product of two matrices, the different suggestions have been made. The most popular composition is a version with the maximum applied instead of the outer sum, and the minimum replaces the inner multiplication.

**Definition 2.11** (max-min composition) [12, 40, 88, 95]

Let $X=\{x_1, \ldots, x_m\}$, $Y=\{y_1, \ldots, y_n\}$ and $Z=\{z_1, \ldots, z_p\}$. We introduce $\widetilde{R}$ with $\mu_{\widetilde{R}}(x_i, y_j)$, $(x_i, y_j)\in X\times Y$, and $\widetilde{Q}$ with $\mu_{\widetilde{Q}}(y_j, z_k)$, $(y_j, z_k)\in Y\times Z$, $i=1, \ldots, m$, $j=1, \ldots, n$, $k=1, \ldots, p$, as two fuzzy relations. The max-min composition of $\widetilde{R}$ with $\widetilde{Q}$, denoted by $\widetilde{R}\circ\widetilde{Q}$, will be a fuzzy relation [12, 40, 95]

$$\tilde{S}=\tilde{R}\circ\tilde{Q}=\left\{\left((x_i, z_k), \mu_{\tilde{R}\circ\tilde{Q}}(x_i, z_k)=\max_{y_j\in Y}\left\{\min\left\{\mu_{\tilde{R}}(x_i, y_j), \mu_{\tilde{Q}}(y_j, z_k)\right\}\right\}\right)\right\}. \quad (2.21)$$

The next example throws more light on the last definition by explaining the meaning of performed operations. In order to introduce the entry data we propose using two rectangular matrices that correspond to two fuzzy relations.

**Example 2.19**

The relation $\widetilde{R}$ reveals via values of membership degrees $\mu_{\widetilde{R}}(x_i, y_j)$, $i = 1, 2$, $j = 1, 2, 3$, the connective dependence between $X$ = "*the intensity of sun radiation*" = $\{x_1$ – "*low radiation*", $x_2$ – "*high radiation*"$\}$ and $Y$ = "*the daily temperature*" = $\{y_1$ – "*the temperature in the morning*", $y_2$ – "*the temperature at noon*", $y_3$ – "*the temperature in the evening*"$\}$. After inserting the membership degrees to each pair of $\widetilde{R}$ we state its content by the matrix

$$\widetilde{R} = \begin{array}{c} \\ x_1 \\ x_2 \end{array}\begin{array}{c} \begin{array}{ccc} y_1 & y_2 & y_3 \end{array} \\ \begin{bmatrix} 0.8 & 0.5 & 0.7 \\ 0.4 & 0.9 & 0.5 \end{bmatrix} \end{array}.$$

The next relation $\widetilde{Q}$ settles the relationship between $Y$ = "*the daily temperature*" represented by $y_1, y_2, y_3$, and two states of $Z$ = "*the moisture of soil*" = $\{z_1$ – "*low moisture*", $z_2$ – "*high moisture*"$\}$. The membership degrees $\mu_{\widetilde{Q}}(y_j, z_k)$, $j = 1, 2, 3$, $k = 1, 2$, express the truthfulness of a connection between $Y$ and $Z$ as

$$\widetilde{Q} = \begin{array}{c} \\ y_1 \\ y_2 \\ y_3 \end{array}\begin{array}{c} \begin{array}{cc} z_1 & z_2 \end{array} \\ \begin{bmatrix} 0.3 & 0.9 \\ 0.8 & 0.3 \\ 0.5 & 0.7 \end{bmatrix} \end{array}.$$

By composing the relations $\widetilde{R}$ and $\widetilde{Q}$ we should obtain the result that reveals the association between $X$ and $Z$ described by the values of membership degrees as follows

$$\widetilde{S} = \begin{array}{c} \\ x_1 \\ x_2 \end{array}\begin{array}{c} \begin{array}{cc} z_1 & z_2 \end{array} \\ \begin{bmatrix} \max(\min(0.8,0.3), \min(0.5,0.8), \min(0.7,0.5)) & \max(\min(0.8,0.9), \min(0.5,0.3), \min(0.7,0.7)) \\ \max(\min(0.4,0.3), \min(0.9,0.8), \min(0.5,0.5)) & \max(\min(0.4,0.9), \min(0.9,0.3), \min(0.5,0.7)) \end{bmatrix} \end{array}$$

$$= \begin{array}{c} \\ x_1 \\ x_2 \end{array}\begin{array}{c} \begin{array}{cc} z_1 & z_2 \end{array} \\ \begin{bmatrix} \max(0.3,0.5,0.5) & \max(0.8,0.3,0.7) \\ \max(0.3,0.8,0.5) & \max(0.4,0.3,0.5) \end{bmatrix} \end{array} = \begin{array}{c} \\ x_1 \\ x_2 \end{array}\begin{array}{c} \begin{array}{cc} z_1 & z_2 \end{array} \\ \begin{bmatrix} 0.5 & 0.8 \\ 0.8 & 0.5 \end{bmatrix} \end{array}.$$

The value 0.8 assigned to the pairs (low radiation, high moisture) and (high radiation, low moisture) seems to confirm a truthful association between the examined parameters "*sun radiation*" and "*soil moisture*". It is also acceptable to admit that the connection between low radiation and low moisture or high radiation and high moisture is appreciated as true in the grade 0.5.

Even this simple example convinces us about the importance of a decisive character of the max-min composition. In spite of the greatest popularity, the results of the operation sometimes are interpreted as too "sharp" because of the action of the inner operation min that causes an essential consideration of the smallest values. To smooth this inconvenient effect, it is suggested to introduce another general definition of the composition of two fuzzy relations.

**Definition 2.12**

Let $\tilde{R}$ and $\tilde{Q}$ be the relations from Def. 2.11. The max-∗ composition of $\tilde{R}$ and $\tilde{Q}$ is now defined as

$$\tilde{R} \underset{*}{\circ} \tilde{Q} = \left\{ \left( (x_i, z_k), \mu_{\tilde{R} \underset{*}{\circ} \tilde{Q}}(x_i, z_k) = \max_{y_j \in Y} \left\{ \mu_{\tilde{R}}(x_i, y_j) * \mu_{\tilde{Q}}(y_j, z_k) \right\} \right) \right\} \tag{2.22}$$

for $x_i \in X, y_j \in Y, z_k \in Z$, where "∗" is an associative operation that is monotonically non-decreasing in each argument [95].

An arbitrary *t*-norm satisfies the conditions of monotonicity and associativity (properties 2. and 4. in (2.11)); therefore it can be utilized in Eq. 2.22. Two special cases of the operation max-∗ are taken into consideration in the following definition.

**Definition 2.13**

Let $\tilde{R}$ and $\tilde{Q}$ be fuzzy relations of the same shape as in Defs 2.11 and 2.12. Hence, the max-*prod* composition $\tilde{R} \underset{\cdot}{\circ} \tilde{Q}$ and the max-*av* composition $\tilde{R} \underset{av}{\circ} \tilde{Q}$ are proposed as fuzzy relations

$$\tilde{R} \underset{\cdot}{\circ} \tilde{Q} = \left\{ \left( (x_i, z_k), \mu_{\tilde{R} \underset{\cdot}{\circ} \tilde{Q}}(x_i, z_k) = \max_{y_j \in Y} \left\{ \mu_{\tilde{R}}(x_i, y_j) \cdot \mu_{\tilde{Q}}(y_j, z_k) \right\} \right) \right\} \tag{2.23}$$

and

$$\tilde{R} \underset{av}{\circ} \tilde{Q} = \left\{ \left( (x_i, z_k), \mu_{\tilde{R} \underset{av}{\circ} \tilde{Q}}(x_i, z_k) = \frac{1}{2} \cdot \max_{y_j \in Y} \left\{ \mu_{\tilde{R}}(x_i, y_j) + \mu_{\tilde{Q}}(y_j, z_k) \right\} \right) \right. \quad (2.24)$$

for $x_i \in X, y_j \in Y, z_k \in Z$ .

The operation $\mu_{\tilde{R}} + \mu_{\tilde{Q}}$ used in (2.24) has not all properties of a $t$-norm but it fulfils the conditions 2. and 4. composed in (2.11). This classifies the sum of membership degrees as the appropriate operation "$*$", accepted in the composition of fuzzy relations [95].

We return to the basic relations $\tilde{R}$ and $\tilde{Q}$ from Ex. 2.19 to test results of the formulas (2.23), (2.24) and to compare these results to the effects of the max-min composition already obtained in Ex. 2.19.

**Example 2.20**

Let us compute the relations $\tilde{R} \circ \tilde{Q}$ and $\tilde{R} \underset{av}{\circ} \tilde{Q}$ for $\tilde{R}$ and $\tilde{Q}$ from Ex. 2.19. By applying Eq. (2.23) we obtain

$$\tilde{R} \circ \tilde{Q} = \begin{array}{c} \\ x_1 \\ x_2 \end{array} \begin{array}{c} \begin{array}{cc} \quad z_1 \quad & \quad z_2 \quad \end{array} \\ \begin{bmatrix} \max(0.8 \cdot 0.3, 0.5 \cdot 0.8, 0.7 \cdot 0.5) & \max(0.8 \cdot 0.9, 0.5 \cdot 0.3, 0.7 \cdot 0.7) \\ \max(0.4 \cdot 0.3, 0.9 \cdot 0.8, 0.5 \cdot 0.5) & \max(0.4 \cdot 0.9, 0.9 \cdot 0.3, 0.5 \cdot 0.7) \end{bmatrix} \end{array}$$

$$= \begin{array}{c} \\ x_1 \\ x_2 \end{array} \begin{array}{c} \begin{array}{cc} \quad z_1 \quad & \quad z_2 \quad \end{array} \\ \begin{bmatrix} \max(0.24, 0.4, 0.35) & \max(0.72, 0.15, 0.49) \\ \max(0.12, 0.72, 0.25) & \max(0.36, 0.27, 0.35) \end{bmatrix} \end{array} = \begin{array}{c} \\ x_1 \\ x_2 \end{array} \begin{array}{c} \begin{array}{cc} z_1 & z_2 \end{array} \\ \begin{bmatrix} 0.4 & 0.72 \\ 0.72 & 0.36 \end{bmatrix} \end{array}$$

while the formula (2.24) used to the max-$av$ composition yields a matrix

$$\tilde{R} \underset{av}{\circ} \tilde{Q} = \begin{array}{c} \\ x_1 \\ x_2 \end{array} \begin{array}{c} \begin{array}{cc} \quad z_1 \quad & \quad z_2 \quad \end{array} \\ \begin{bmatrix} \frac{1}{2} \cdot \max(0.8 + 0.3, 0.5 + 0.8, 0.7 + 0.5) & \frac{1}{2} \cdot \max(0.8 + 0.9, 0.5 + 0.3, 0.7 + 0.7) \\ \frac{1}{2} \cdot \max(0.4 + 0.3, 0.9 + 0.8, 0.5 + 0.5) & \frac{1}{2} \cdot \max(0.4 + 0.9, 0.9 + 0.3, 0.5 + 0.7) \end{bmatrix} \end{array}$$

$$
= \begin{array}{c} \\ x_1 \\ \\ x_2 \end{array}
\begin{array}{cc} z_1 & z_2 \end{array}
\begin{bmatrix} \frac{1}{2}\cdot\max(1.1,1.3,1.2) & \frac{1}{2}\cdot\max(1.7,0.8,1.4) \\ \frac{1}{2}\cdot\max(0.7,1.7,1.0) & \frac{1}{2}\cdot\max(1.3,1.2,1.2) \end{bmatrix}
= \begin{array}{c} x_1 \\ x_2 \end{array}
\begin{bmatrix} 0.65 & 0.85 \\ 0.85 & 0.65 \end{bmatrix}.
$$

where the columns of both matrices are labelled $z_1$, $z_2$.

By analyzing the results of three tested operations $\tilde{R}\circ\tilde{Q}$, $\tilde{R}\underset{\cdot}{\circ}\tilde{Q}$ and $\tilde{R}\underset{av}{\circ}\tilde{Q}$, we conclude that it would be the most reliable to choose the second composition $\tilde{R}\underset{\cdot}{\circ}\tilde{Q}$ in further medical investigations. The choice is justified by the fact that the difference between two essential stages (*high radiation*, *high moisture*) and (*high radiation*, *low moisture*) is emphasized in the remarkable way in the composition $\tilde{R}\underset{\cdot}{\circ}\tilde{Q}$.

In some special cases, when $X = \{x_1\}$, the relation $\tilde{R}$ becomes a one row-relation. Definition 2.13 thus takes the following modified version.

**Definition 2.14**

Let $X = \{x_1\}$, $Y = \{y_1, \ldots, y_n\}$, $Z = \{z_1, \ldots, z_p\}$. We set fuzzy relations $\tilde{R}$ with $\mu_{\tilde{R}}(x_1, y_j)$, $(x_1, y_j) \in X \times Y$ and $\tilde{Q}$ characterized by $\mu_{\tilde{Q}}(y_j, z_k)$, $(y_j, z_k) \in Y \times Z$. The max-*prod* composition of $\tilde{R}$ with $\tilde{Q}$, denoted by $\tilde{R}\underset{\cdot}{\circ}\tilde{Q}$, is a one row fuzzy set

$$
\tilde{R}\underset{\cdot}{\circ}\tilde{Q} = \left\{ \left( (x_1, z_k), \mu_{\tilde{R}\circ\tilde{Q}}(x_1, z_k) = \max_{y_j \in Y} \left\{ \mu_{\tilde{R}}(x_1, y_j) \cdot \mu_{\tilde{Q}}(y_j, z_k) \right\} \right) \right\} \tag{2.25}
$$

for $x_1 \in X, y_j \in Y, z_k \in Z$.

The short and simple introduction that has been accomplished in this chapter is necessary to lead to a further discussion about different mathematical fuzzy models. The models are fitted for the same objective, namely, how to extract different concepts and properties developed by fuzzy set theory in order to transform them to facilitate solutions to medical problems.

# 3 Medical Diagnosis

## 3.1 Introduction

The creators of fuzzy set theory, who develop mathematical models applied to different technical domains, have also made representative contributions in medical investigations. One of the earliest models created by Sanchez [72, 73] and discussed by other scientists [6, 8, 11, 17, 27, 45, 48, 56, 69, 70, 74, 75, 76, 77, 87] has given some answers to questions concerning a choice of diagnosis. The choice should only be made on the basis of clinical symptoms when assuming that the symptoms are typical of all considered diagnoses.

To decide an appropriate diagnosis in one patient we introduce three non-fuzzy sets:

the set of symptoms $S = \{S_1, S_2, ..., S_n\}$,

the set of diagnoses $D = \{D_1, D_2, ..., D_p\}$,

the set of patients $P = \{P_1\}$.

The symptoms occurring in set $S$ are associated with the diagnoses from set $D$. Moreover, we assume that information about all symptoms belonging to $S$ is complete in the patient's case. By using his medical experience as a foundation a physician then establishes connections between the symptoms and the diagnoses.

## 3.2 The Modus Ponens Law in Medical Diagnosis

The symptoms $S_1$, $S_2$, ..., $S_n$, that are stated in set $S$, are included in the pairs $(P_1, S_1)$, $(P_1, S_2)$, ..., $(P_1, S_n)$. These constitute the relation $PS$ ("*patient – symptom*"). Let us write down the fuzzy relation $PS$ as a one-row matrix

$$PS = P_1 \overset{\quad S_1 \qquad\qquad\quad S_2 \qquad \cdots \qquad S_n}{[\mu_{PS}(P_1,S_1) \; \mu_{PS}(P_1,S_2) \cdots \mu_{PS}(P_1,S_n)]}, \tag{3.1}$$

where $\mu_{PS}(P_1, S_j)$, $j = 1, ..., n$, is a value of the membership degree providing us with evaluation of the intensity of $S_j$ in $P_1$.

The next relation consists of the pairs $(S_1, D_1)$, $(S_1, D_2)$, ..., $(S_1, D_p)$, ..., $(S_n, D_p)$. The fuzzy relation, in which each value of the membership degree tied to the pair $(S_j, D_k)$, $j = 1, 2, ..., n$, $k = 1, 2, ..., p$, expresses strength of the relationship

Elisabeth Rakus-Andersson: *Fuzzy and Rough Techniques in Medical Diagnosis and Medication*, StudFuzz **212**, 31–61 (2007)
www.springerlink.com

between the symptom and the associated diagnosis, is called "*symptom – diagnosis*". The relation has the name *SD* and is projected as a matrix

$$SD = \begin{array}{c} \\ S_1 \\ S_2 \\ \vdots \\ S_n \end{array} \begin{array}{c} \begin{array}{cccc} D_1 & D_2 & \cdots & D_p \end{array} \\ \begin{bmatrix} \mu_{SD}(S_1,D_1) & \mu_{SD}(S_1,D_2) & \cdots & \mu_{SD}(S_1,D_p) \\ \mu_{SD}(S_2,D_1) & \mu_{SD}(S_2,D_2) & \cdots & \mu_{SD}(S_2,D_p) \\ \vdots & \vdots & \ddots & \vdots \\ \mu_{SD}(S_n,D_1) & \mu_{SD}(S_n,D_2) & \cdots & \mu_{SD}(S_n,D_p) \end{bmatrix} \end{array}. \tag{3.2}$$

In the further discussion we suppose that the relation *PS* is generally interpreted as a statement

"*p*" = "the symptoms $S_j$, $j = 1, 2, \ldots, n$, are found in patient $P_1$".

The relation *SD* stands for an implication

"*p*′ IMPLIES *q*" = "the symptoms $S_j$ confirm presence of the diagnoses $D_k$ (if $S_j$ then $D_k$), $j = 1, 2, \ldots, n$, $k = 1, 2, \ldots, p$".

The statement *p*′ is nearly the same as *p*, but these two sentences *p* and *p*′ do not need to be worded identically.

By quoting the rule *modus ponens*

IF "*p*" AND "*p*′ IMPLIES *q*" THEN *q*′"

we expect getting the conclusion

"*q*′"= "the diagnoses $D_k$, $k = 1, 2, \ldots, p$, are assigned to $P_1$".

As the result of the last sentence *q*′ a relation *PD* has been produced. The *PD* ("*patient – diagnosis*") relation is a matrix

$$\begin{array}{c} \qquad\quad D_1 \qquad\qquad D_2 \qquad \cdots \qquad D_p \\ PD = P_1[\mu_{PD}(P_1,D_1)\ \mu_{PD}(P_1,D_2)\ \cdots\ \mu_{PD}(P_1,D_p)], \end{array} \tag{3.3}$$

in which the membership degrees reveal associations between the patient and the diagnoses.

To make a proper choice of the diagnosis that is the most applicable for the examined patient when regarding his or her symptoms, we employ the *modus ponens* rule as follows.

**Definition 3.1**

If the premise "the symptoms $S_j$, $j = 1, 2, \ldots, n$, are found in patient $P_1$" is given by the relation *PS*, and the hypothesis "the symptoms $S_j$ imply the diagnoses $D_k$, $j = 1, 2, \ldots, n$, $k = 1, 2, \ldots, p$" is represented by the relation *SD*, then the relation $PD = PS \circ SD$, formed as a result of the thesis "$P_1$ suffers from $D_k$", will be composed of membership degrees allowing us to estimate associations between the patient and the considered diagnoses.

We will study some modifications of Def. 3.1 in the next subsections.

## 3.3 The *Patient –Symptom* Relation

Each symptom belonging to the set *S* will be represented as a fuzzy set.

We adopt three basic types of biological parameters [29, 30, 32, 56]:

1. Simple qualitative features,
2. Compound qualitative features,
3. Quantitative (measurable) features.

**Example 3.1**

Suppose that symptoms from set *S*, characteristic of $P_1$, are listed as: $S_1$ – "*hereditary inclination*", $S_2$ – "*ECG changes in resting position*", $S_3$ – "*smoking*", $S_4$ – "*lack of physical activity*", $S_5$ – "*pain in chest*", $S_6$ –"*breathlessness*", $S_7$ – "*feeling of sickness*", $S_8$ – "*hypertension*", $S_9$ – "*increased level of LDL-cholesterol*", $S_{10}$ – "*obesity*".

By studying the nature of the symptoms we can divide them into three following groups:

1. $S_1$ is interpreted as the simple qualitative feature that is present or lacking;
2. $S_2$, $S_3$, $S_4$, $S_5$, $S_6$, $S_7$ are investigated with the help of a questionnaire as compound qualitative symptoms;
3. $S_8$, $S_9$, $S_{10}$ are typical measurable parameters that are described by values obtained in examinations carried out.

Since every symptom is considered as a fuzzy set then we should decide the set's support and values of membership degrees assigned to the members of the support. The ways of membership degree constructions should reflect intensities of symptoms acting as important indications of the patient's health.

We now intend to concentrate this discussion on three types of symptoms that will be designed as fuzzy sets. Since they represent different features then we will be obliged to invent varying methods of designing membership functions for them.

### 3.3.1 Simple Qualitative Biological Parameters

The fuzzy set characterizing this symptom is defined in a space {0, 1}. If the symptom $S_j$ does not occur in the patient, the number 0 will symbolize its lack. It means that element $x$ of the fuzzy set $S_j$ takes the value 0, and the membership degree of this element is fixed to be 0, too.

If the symptom $S_j$ is found in the patient, we agree to note this fact down as the number 1. Thus, element $x$ takes the value 1 and the membership degree of $x$ is also determined as 1.

The fuzzy set $S_j$ corresponding to the symptom $S_j$ is often written down symbolically as

$$S_j = {}^{0}\!/_{0} + {}^{1}\!/_{1} . \tag{3.4}$$

In Eq. (3.4) both the symptom and the fuzzy set representing it have the same denotation in order not to introduce too many symbols.

**Example 3.2**

Suppose that patient $P_1$ has had relatives who have suffered from cardiovascular system diseases. Hence, his tendency to inherit these diseases is evaluated as $x = 1$ and $S_1(1) = 1$. Consequently, the value of $S_1(1) = 1$ takes also its place in the relation $PS$ that is actualized as

$$PS = P_1 \begin{array}{c} \\ \left[ \right. \end{array} \begin{array}{cccccccccc} S_1 & S_2 & S_3 & S_4 & S_5 & S_6 & S_7 & S_8 & S_9 & S_{10} \\ 1 & & & & & & & & & \end{array} \begin{array}{c} \\ \left. \right] \end{array} .$$

The qualitative attribute wearing the simple complexity is the simplest possible. It is frequently required to have a wider approach to the ascertainment of qualitative features, for example, by applying a questionnaire with questions and alternative answers to the questions being posed. This is designed in the case of compound qualitative features for which the construction of fuzzy set $S_j$ corresponding to the symptom $S_j$ is thoroughly explained below.

### 3.3.2 Compound Qualitative Biological Features

We assume now that the symptom $S_j$ is no longer determined by one of the alternatives "*present* – *absent*", but it needs a certain verbal description. Let us introduce a new variable supporting $S_j$, the linguistic variable $Q^{S(j)}$, with the set of terms formed by the questions (asked by a physician or by a questionnaire) that are denoted here by $q_p^{S(j)}$, $p = 1, 2, \ldots, Q^{S(j)-last\,question}$ [29, 30, 32, 56, 70]. The symbol $Q^{S(j)\text{-}last\ question}$ stands for the quantity of questions associated with the symbol $S_j$.

To each of the questions $q_p^{S(j)}$ posed to the person being examined in connection with the symptom $S_j$ found, he/she has a possibility of choosing one of several answers that are usually furnished with numbers-codes $s_{p,t}^{S(j)} = 0,1,2, \ldots, N$, $p = 1,2, \ldots, Q^{S(j)-last\,question}$, $t = 1,2, \ldots, t^{(p)}$. The symbol $t^{(p)}$ designates the number of alternative answers to the question $q_p^{S(j)}$, and we understand that the value $t = 1$ is connected to the choice of the code "0", while $t = t^{(p)}$ must be associated with pointing to the code "$N$". The codes 0, 1, …, $N$ are hierarchical replacements of the answers from the most negative (denying the presence of $S_j$) to the most positive (confirming the existence of the symptom).

In the further procedure, one should assign weights $w_{p,t}^{S(j)}$ to the encoded (proposed) answers $s_{p,t}^{S(j)}$ [70]. These weights are suggested to be numbers belonging to the interval [–1, 1]. It is assumed that negative numbers correspond to negative answers to the question posed, i.e., ones that do not confirm the occurrence of the symptom (never, rarely, very rarely and the like), with that –1 defines the most negative answer. The positive value of the weight gives a suitable positive character, certifying the presence of the symptom in the patient, and the value +1 confirms the entire presence of the symptom. The weight equal to zero (or close to zero) is reserved for the case of the lack of the answer or a statement that does not bring any (or almost any) information.

The set of questions in $Q^{S(j)}$ is treated as a list of terms representing the linguistic variable $Q^{S(j)}$. Each question $q_p^{S(j)}$, $p = 1,2, \ldots, Q^{S(j)-last\,question}$, is interpreted as a fuzzy variable with the support, established via weights, equal to [–1, 1]. This conception helps to build a fuzzy set $S_j$ reflecting the compound qualitative symptom $S_j$ with the same name.

The value of a weight lying in the subintervals [–1, 0] and [0, 1], respectively, depends on the number of a code 1, 2, …, $N$, chosen by the patient who answers a corresponding question. The above-mentioned intervals are, in general, decomposed evenly according to the number of alternative answers. The endpoints of the subintervals thus formed constitute the values of the weights for all the alternative answers. The number of the weights is finite and equal, as a rule, to a slight number of answers. To represent the symptom $S_j$ by one value being a result of an operation concatenating all weights assigned to the questions $q_p^{S(j)}$, $p$ = 1, 2, …, $Q^{S(j)-last\,question}$, it seems to be purposeful to bring into use a continuous aggregation function.

To sum up, let $S_j$ be the fuzzy set for a compound qualitative feature. This set is fully defined when both its support and its membership function is given. The function should be, in turn, considered in a real space $X$ and built as a set of weight aggregation results. Therefore it is essential to transpose the qualitative feature to measurable values, i.e., to values $x$ belonging to $X$, where $X$ is regarded as a support of $S_j$. To concatenate the weights of all answers as a common value $x$ describing $S_j$, we suggest the mapping

$$x = \sum_{p=1}^{Q^{S(j)-last\,question}} w_{p,t}^{S(j)} . \tag{3.5}$$

The operation means the addition of the weights determined for the answers to the questions that collect information about $S_j$ (every question is represented by only one weight joined to the alternative answer $t = 1, \ldots, t^{(p)}$).

The values of $x$ form an interval bounded below by some number $\alpha$ that is calculated from the formula

$$\alpha = \sum_{p=1}^{Q^{S(j)-last\,question}} \min_{1 \le t \le t^{(p)}} (w_{p,t}^{S(j)}) , \tag{3.6}$$

i.e., is assumed to be the sum of the weights, smallest as far as their relative values are concerned, assigned to the most negative answers to each question giving a picture of $S_j$.

A number $\gamma$ bounds this interval from above and is fixed in accordance with the equation

$$\gamma = \sum_{p=1}^{Q^{S(j)-last\,question}} \max_{1 \le t \le t^{(p)}} (w_{p,t}^{S(j)}) \tag{3.7}$$

that means that one should calculate the sum of the weights greatest as far as their relative values are concerned. They are quantities representing the extreme positive answers to the questions concerning the symptom $S_j$.

The conclusions, implied above, have led to the construction of the support of the compound qualitative attribute $S_j$ defined as the interval $[\alpha, \gamma]$. The membership function over $[\alpha, \gamma]$ is put forward for consideration as [29, 30, 32, 56]

$$y = \mu_{S_j}(x) = s(x, \alpha, \beta, \gamma) , \tag{3.8}$$

in which $s(x, \alpha, \beta, \gamma)$ is given by Eq. (2.5).

**Example 3.3**

If a value of the weight assigned to the extreme negative answer is fixed at $-1$ and the weight of its most positive variant is equal to $+1$, and the rule is preserved for each question, then the graph of the function (3.8), designed for five questions characteristic of $S_j$ and formed as the equation $y = \mu_{S_j}(x) = s(x, -5, 0, 5)$, will take the symmetrical form as given in Fig. 3.1.

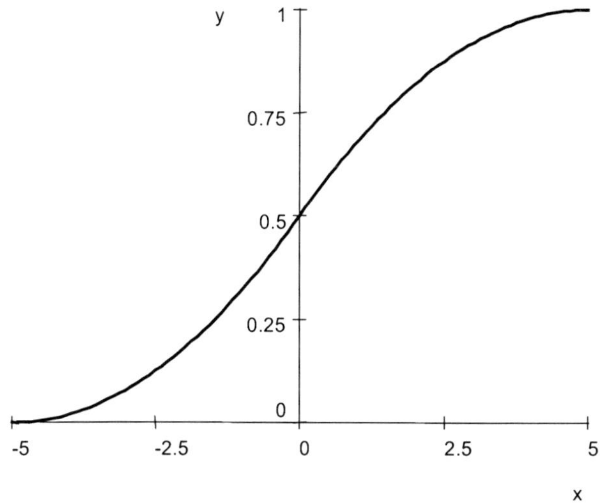


Figure 3.1: The membership function of the compound qualitative symptom $S_j$

By analysing the graph we can notice there the number $\alpha = -5$. That is the sum of the minimal weights representing the five answers negating the symptom presence, it has the assigned membership degree equal to zero. This is a sign of "health". The number $\gamma = 5$ is a sum of maximally positive weights confirming the revealed symptom and, in consequence, the membership degree associated with it takes the value 1. An ambiguous piece of information or its lack, expressed by $\beta$, has its mapping in the form of the membership degree of the value 0.5.

To illustrate the action of computing the membership degrees for compound qualitative symptoms, let us state the values of degrees for some of the symptoms of this character found in patient $P_1$, with whom we have already made an acquaintance in Ex. 3.1.

**Example 3.4**

By composing a questionnaire, which yields the information of intensity accompanying the symptoms $S_3$ and $S_4$, we assign the membership degree to each of them.

An inquiry of the first considered symptom $S_3$ – "*smoking*", is accomplished by answering questions, e.g.:

$q_1^{S(3)}$ ="*How often do you smoke cigarettes?*"

$q_2^{S(3)}$ ="*How long have you smoked?*"

The alternative answers to these questions may be formulated, for instance, as follows:

– to the first question $q_1^{S(3)}$

1. *I do not smoke* $s_{1,1}^{S(3)} = 0$ $w_{1,1}^{S(3)} = -1$
2. *I smoke seldom* $s_{1,2}^{S(3)} = 1$ $w_{1,2}^{S(3)} = -\frac{1}{2}$
3. *I smoke moderately* $s_{1,3}^{S(3)} = 2$ $w_{1,3}^{S(3)} = 0$
4. *I smoke often* $s_{1,4}^{S(3)} = 3$ $w_{1,4}^{S(3)} = \frac{1}{2}$
5. *I smoke constantly* $s_{1,5}^{S(3)} = 4$ $w_{1,5}^{S(3)} = 1$

– to the second question $q_2^{S(3)}$

1. *I have never smoked* $s_{2,1}^{S(3)} = 0$ $w_{2,1}^{S(3)} = -1$
2. *A few months* $s_{2,2}^{S(3)} = 1$ $w_{2,2}^{S(3)} = -\frac{2}{3}$
3. *1–2 years* $s_{2,3}^{S(3)} = 2$ $w_{2,3}^{S(3)} = -\frac{1}{3}$
4. *I cannot determine* $s_{2,4}^{S(3)} = 3$ $w_{2,4}^{S(3)} = 0$
5. *3–4 years* $s_{2,5}^{S(3)} = 4$ $w_{2,5}^{S(3)} = \frac{1}{3}$
6. *More than 5 years* $s_{2,6}^{S(3)} = 5$ $w_{2,6}^{S(3)} = \frac{2}{3}$
7. *I have smoked since my teens* $s_{2,7}^{S(3)} = 6$ $w_{2,7}^{S(3)} = 1$ .

We assume that patient $P_1$ has chosen answer *4.* to $q_1^{S(3)}$ and answer *6.* to $q_2^{S(3)}$; hence, $x = \frac{1}{2} + \frac{2}{3} = \frac{7}{6}$, $\alpha = (-1) + (-1) = -2$, $\gamma = 1 + 1 = 2$, $\beta = 0$, and

$\mu_{S_3}(x) = s(x,-2,0,2) = 1 - 2\left(\frac{x-2}{2-(-2)}\right)^2$ in view of $x > 0$, that is $\mu_{S_3}\left(\frac{7}{6}\right) \approx 0.913$ .

The pair ($P_1$, $S_3$) of the relation *PS* has therefore the membership degree equal to 0.913. This degree characterizes a feature such as "*smoking*" efficiently, since it reflects every subtle distinction in the patient's report when comparing the extreme information of the type "*I smoke*" contrary to "*I do not smoke*".

The other parameter $S_4$ – "*lack of physical activity*" can be described, as an instance, by three questions:

$q_1^{S(4)}$ = "*Do you sometimes exercise?*"

$q_2^{S(4)}$ = "*How intensively do you exercise?*"

$q_3^{S(4)}$ = "*How long have you exercised?*"

The answers proposed in the questionnaire with their codes and weights are established as:

– to the first question $q_1^{S(4)}$

1. *I exercise every day* $w_{1,1}^{S(4)} = -1$
2. *I exercise often* $w_{1,2}^{S(4)} = -\frac{1}{2}$
3. *I cannot say* $w_{1,3}^{S(4)} = 0$
4. *I exercise little* $w_{1,4}^{S(4)} = \frac{1}{2}$
5. *I do not exercise* $w_{1,5}^{S(4)} = 1$

– to the second question $q_2^{S(4)}$

1. *I exercise very hard* $w_{2,1}^{S(4)} = -1$
2. *I exercise rather hard* $w_{2,2}^{S(4)} = -\frac{1}{2}$
3. *It is difficult to say* $w_{2,3}^{S(4)} = 0$
4. *I do light exercises* $w_{2,4}^{S(4)} = \frac{1}{2}$
5. *I do not do any exercises* $w_{2,5}^{S(4)} = 1$

– to the third question $q_3^{S(4)}$

1. *I have exercised since my teens* $w_{3,1}^{S(4)} = -1$
2. *More than 5 years* $w_{3,2}^{S(4)} = -\frac{2}{3}$
3. *3–4 years* $w_{3,3}^{S(4)} = -\frac{1}{3}$
4. *I cannot determine* $w_{3,4}^{S(4)} = 0$
5. *1–2 years* $w_{3,5}^{S(4)} = \frac{1}{3}$
6. *A few months* $w_{3,6}^{S(4)} = \frac{2}{3}$
7. *I have never exercised* $w_{3,7}^{S(4)} = 1$.

Let us notice that the lack of *exercising* is regarded as a harmful symptom for some diseases. This is expressed by assigning the positive values of weights to the answers that confirm the bad physical condition. On the contrary, a well-trained person does not run a great risk of falling ill. Exercising can increase the health condition and therefore is added to prior physical factors. The answers pointing to a good physical form have thus the negative weights attached.

If patient $P_1$ marks the answers *3. 4.* and *4.*, respectively, we should find the value of the element $x$ for $S_4$ as $x = 0 + \frac{1}{2} + 0 = \frac{1}{2}$, $\alpha = (-1) + (-1) + (-1) = -3$, $\gamma = 1 + 1 + 1 = 3$, $\beta = 0$, and $\mu_{S_4}(x) = s(x, -3, 0, 3) = 1 - 2\left(\frac{x-3}{3-(-3)}\right)^2$ because of the positive value of $x$ that gives $\mu_{S_4}\left(\frac{1}{2}\right) \approx 0.653$.

The compound qualitative attribute $S_4$ has been assessed by the value of the membership degree 0.653. We act in the same way as discussed above to state the membership degrees of the rest of the compound qualitative attributes, calculating them as, e.g.,

$\mu_{S_2 - \text{"ECG changes in resting position"}}(x) = 0.515$,

$\mu_{S_5 - \text{"pain in chest"}}(x) = 0.345$,

$\mu_{S_6 - \text{"breathnessless"}}(x) = 0.632$,

$\mu_{S_7 - \text{"feeling of sickness"}}(x) = 0.720$.

The values of $x$ via weights characterize the questionnaire answers of patient $P_1$. The membership degrees of $x$ fill up some remaining empty positions in the relation *PS*. After completing the missing values the relation *PS* has its content presented as

$$\begin{array}{lcccccccccc} & S_1 & S_2 & S_3 & S_4 & S_5 & S_6 & S_7 & S_8 & S_9 & S_{10} \\ PS = P_1[ & 1 & 0.515 & 0.913 & 0.653 & 0.345 & 0.632 & 0.720 & & & ]. \end{array}$$

There still exist three symptoms $S_8$, $S_9$ and $S_{10}$ that do not have their membership degrees determined. The mentioned parameters belong to the third symptom class created for quantitative features. To find their membership values we refer to "arguing", which is portrayed in the next subsection.

### 3.3.3 Compound Quantitative Biological Features

A quantitative (measurable) feature is the last type of a biological parameter for which a model of defining the membership degree in the relation *PS* has been produced. These features take values continuously from a known interval determined by a physician. The measurable symptom $S_j$ can be represented as the fuzzy set $S_j$ with values from the interval containing all possible quantities taken by this feature. We denote this interval by [*VMIN*, *VMAX*] with the notations; *VMIN* is the minimal value taken by the parameter and, respectively, *VMAX* is its maximal value. Let us give the symbols $VN_1$, $VN_2$ to the limits of the interval in which there occur numbers characteristic of healthy man. It should be noticed that, outside the interval ($VN_1$, $VN_2$), both the deficiency and the excess of a biological indicator is a disease sign, most frequently connected with different diagnoses. Therefore one should divide the interval [*VMIN*, *VMAX*] adopted originally and write it down as [29, 30, 32, 56]

$$[VMIN, VMAX] = [VMIN, VN_1] \cup (VN_1, VN_2) \cup [VN_2, VMAX]. \tag{3.9}$$

The membership function of the set $S_j$, defined on the interval (3.9) ought to express reliably all disease states examined on the basis on the symptom $S_j$. For symptoms whose uniform growth of values is connected with a uniformly progressing disease, one proposes the membership function

$$y = \mu_{S_j}(x) = \begin{cases} s\left(x, VN_2, \dfrac{VN_2 + VMAX}{2}, VMAX\right) & \text{for} \quad VN_2 \le x \le VMAX, \\ 0 & \text{for} \quad VN_1 < x < VN_2, \\ 1 - s\left(x, VMIN, \dfrac{VMIN + VN_1}{2}, VN_1\right) & \text{for} \quad VMIN \le x \le VN_1, \end{cases} \tag{3.10}$$

where $x$ stands for the value taken by $S_j$.

**Example 3.5**

The quantitative symptom $S_8$ – "*hypertension*" from Ex. 3.1 is a consequence of increased values of systolic blood pressure. This parameter has an interval of normal values, typical of a healthy man, established as ($VN_1$, $VN_2$) = (90 *mmHg*, 120 *mmHg*) while *VMIN*, *VMAX* are appreciated as 50 *mmHg*, 250 *mmHg*, respectively. It is worth mentioning that high values of systolic blood pressure are assigned – as warning signals – to cardiovascular diseases. Opposite to it, very low values of systolic blood pressure are typical of, e.g., acute bleeding. On the condition that the membership function of $S_8$ reflects a uniformly progressive sickly state, we propose to explore it by the equation

$$y = \mu_{S_8}(x) = \begin{cases} s\left(x, 120, \dfrac{120 + 250}{2}, 250\right) & \text{for} \quad 120 \le x \le 250, \\ 0 & \text{for} \quad 90 < x < 120, \\ 1 - s\left(x, 50, \dfrac{50 + 90}{2}, 90\right) & \text{for} \quad 50 \le x \le 90, \end{cases}$$

represented by the graph displayed in Fig. 3.2.

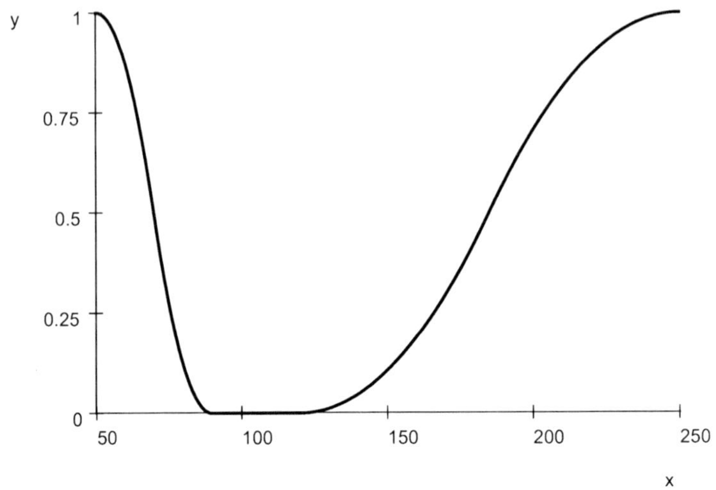


Figure 3.2: The membership function of the symptom $S_8$

More complicated medical phenomena can be divided into two following groups. The physician often finds that the growth of a value characterizing the symptom and belonging to the interval $[VN_2, VMAX]$ (or to $[VMIN, VN_1]$ when the value is lowered instead) does not matter essentially till some moment, and only a high level of the indicator is connected with a violent deterioration of the health condition.

Then it would be purposeful to apply a concentration operation CON for the membership function of the fuzzy set $S_j$ over the interval $[VN_2, VMAX]$ (or $[VMIN, VN_1]$), that is, to use the membership function of the type

$$y = \mu_{CON(S_j)}(x) = \left(\mu_{(S_j)}(x)\right)^2 . \tag{3.11}$$

Conversely, if the physician describes that what constitutes the greatest danger for one's health is the growth of the symptom value at the first stage, then it is advisable to introduce a dilution operation DIL for the symptom $S_j$ that changes the membership function $\mu_{S_j}(x)$ in the following manner

$$y = \mu_{DIL(S_j)}(x) = \sqrt{\mu_{S_j}(x)} . \tag{3.12}$$

The membership function of $S_j$ modified by (3.11) or (3.12) better reflects the patient's physical state when an irregular development of the symptom $S_j$ has an importance in finding the appropriate diagnosis.

**Example 3.6**

The graphs of the function (3.10) as well as the above-described tendencies towards a reliable adoption of the membership function for a measurable feature $S_8$, discussed in Ex. 3.5, are shown in Fig. 3.3.

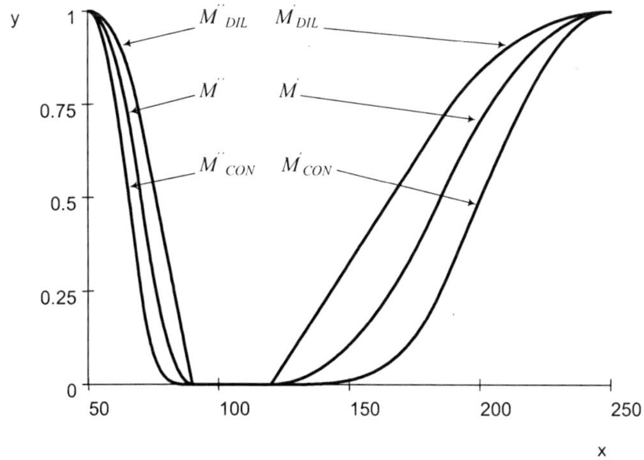


Figure 3.3: The membership function of the symptom $S_8$ with modifications

In the description of the figure we have adopted the notations

$$M' = s\left(x, 120, \frac{120+250}{2}, 250\right) \quad \text{for} \quad 120 \le x \le 250,$$

$$M'' = 1 - s\left(x, 50, \frac{50+90}{2}, 90\right) \quad \text{for} \quad 50 \le x \le 90.$$

The results of Eqs (3.11) and (3.12) obtained in the form of modified membership degrees, in comparison to the effects of (3.10), are intended to be treated as reliable indicators of the symptom's decisive effect on a diagnosis choice.

**Example 3.7**

The physician decides that the value of $S_8$, found in $P_1$, is equal to 210 *mmHg* and points to a severe state of the patient's health. We expect that an appropriate membership degree will be associated with the value of $S_8$ in order to indicate the essential impendence of $P_1$'s health. To start the computations, we choose the first part of the function $\mu_{S_8}(x)$ from Ex. 3.5 because we notice that the value of $x = 210$ belongs to the interval [120, 250].

Hence,

$$\mu_{S_8}(210) = s\left(210, 120, \frac{120+250}{2}, 250\right) = s(210,120,185,250) =$$

$$1-2\left(\frac{210-250}{250-120}\right)^2 \approx 0.81 .$$

To focus on the essentially heightened blood pressure value of $x = 210$, which convinces us that the patient's health is in danger, we should increase $\mu_{S_8}(210)$ by adopting the dilution operation as $\mu_{DIL(S_8)}(210) = \sqrt{\mu_{S_8}(210)} \approx \sqrt{0.81} = 0.9$ .

It is worth noticing that we should use the third part of the formula derived in Ex. 3.5, i.e., $\mu_{S_j}(x) = 1 - s\left(x, 50, \frac{50+90}{2}, 90\right)$ if the value of systolic blood pressure is less than 90 in any patient. It can happen when the patient meets with violent bleeding. The lower values of systolic blood pressure than the quantities placed in [90, 120] characterize another symptom that differs from $S_8$.

The growth of *LDL*-cholesterol also informs a physician about a worse condition of the examined patient. To accentuate the importance of the increased level of $S_9$ – "*increased level of LDL-cholesterol*" we try to generate a reliable value of its membership degree in *PS*.

**Example 3.8**

By carrying out *LDL-cholesterol* level examinations in $P_1$, the physician has established the value of $S_9$ as 145 *mg*/*dl*. If he also decides the values of *VMIN* = 50 *mg*/*dl*, *VMAX* = 250 *mg*/*dl* and states the interval ($VN_1$, $VN_2$) as (100 *mg*/*dl*, 135 *mg*/*dl*), then we are capable of assigning the membership degree of $x = 145$ in accordance with the first "branch" of the membership function given by (3.10) as $\mu_{S_9}(145) = s(145, 135, 192.5, 250) = 2\left(\frac{145-135}{250-135}\right)^2 \approx 0.02$ . Since the value of $x =$ 145 does not lay emphasis on any greater threat for $P_1$'s health, then we should lower the value of the membership degree for the $x$-number. We will reduce it if we apply the concentration operation (3.11) in the form of $\mu_{CON(S_9)}(145)$ $= \left(\mu_{S_9}(145)\right)^2 \approx 0.0004$ .

By using these similar techniques on the symptom $S_{10}$, we assign to its missing representative, in the relation *PS*, the value of the membership degree decided as $\mu_{S_{10}-\text{"obesity"}}(x) = 0.353$, when measuring "*weight*" = 115 *kg* in relation to "*height*" = 1.80 *m*. The grade of obesity $x$ is determined by applying the body mass index $x$ = *BMI* computed as a quotient "*body weight*/(*body height in meters*)$^2$" in units equal to $kg/m^2$. By taking $x = 35.5\ kg/m^2$, $VMIN = 12\ kg/m^2$, $VMAX = 50\ kg/m^2$, $VN_1 = 18\ kg/m^2$ and $VN_2 = 25\ kg/m^2$ as the parameters' values in

(3.10), we confirm the result 0.353 as the membership degree of $S_{10}$, provided that the growth of body weight has the uniform meaning in the diagnostic decision.

Possessing all the values of the membership degrees for the symptoms listed in Ex. 3.1, we finally complete the matrix *PS* and save it to further computations as

$$\begin{array}{cccccccccccc} & & S_1 & S_2 & S_3 & S_4 & S_5 & S_6 & S_7 & S_8 & S_9 & S_{10} \\ PS = & P_1[ & 1 & 0.515 & 0.913 & 0.653 & 0.345 & 0.632 & 0.720 & 0.9 & 0.0004 & 0.353\ ]. \end{array}$$

The next stage in our investigations is to prepare the matrix *SD* introduced by (3.2) that constitutes the other factor (besides *PS*) in the decision equation $PD = PS \circ SD$.

## 3.4 The *Symptom – Diagnosis* Relation

A mathematical process of developing the forms of associations among the symptoms $S_j$, $j = 1, 2, \ldots, n$, and diagnoses $D_k$, $k = 1, 2, \ldots, p$, constitutes another important task to be fulfilled in the diagnostic problem posed. The connection between $S_j$ and $D_k$ in each pair $(S_j, D_k)$ is rendered as a value of the membership degree accompanied by this pair. The membership degree, in turn, expresses the signification of symptom $S_j$ for diagnosis $D_k$. To determine the intensity of the symptom influence on the diagnosis decisive character, a physician asks two essential questions, namely [2, 3]:

1. How often is $S_j$ found in $D_k$?
2. How often is $S_j$ decisive for $D_k$?

The physician uses his experience to answer the questions by selecting verbal expressions that are included in a certain list. We, by following his advice, concentrate on replacing the chosen word by an appropriate number. To begin with, let us first decide the terms of a common list identically constructed for "*presence*" and "*decisive character*". We decide "*presence*" = "*decisive character*" ={"*never*", "*almost never*", "*very seldom*", "*seldom*", "*rather seldom*", "*moderately*", "*rather often*", "*often*", "*very often*", "*almost always*", "*always*"}. By employing the membership functions (the constraints) of fuzzy variables that correspond to the expressions collected above, we will try to find these membership degrees of the variables that represent them in the most adequate way.

Some suggestions referring to the constraints imposed on fuzzy variables have already been made in Ex. 2.15, but we should honestly admit that the borders of the restrictions proposed there have been chosen empirically rather than by involving any computation technique. There exists a domain in fuzzy set theory that deals with computing with words. Within this field we can mathematically modify some sophisticated linguistic expressions coming from basic verbal items. The supports of fuzzy variables and the membership functions laid over them thus will be elaborated without guessing their values, which seems to improve a correctness of further computations.

### 3.4.1 Numerical Representations of Linguistic Variables

One of the most important features of fuzzy set theory, which makes it very attractive for applications, is its potential for the modelling of natural language expressions. Most works done on this topic focus on some parts of natural language, mostly those that correspond to the so-called "*evaluating linguistic expressions*", i.e., the dissertations show how to build fuzzy constraints for the expressions that mark characteristic limits on an ordered scale [40, 49, 90, 91, 92, 93, 94, 95].

Keeping in mind the premises from Subsection 2.4, let us preserve a reference set as the range $A = [0, A_l]$. This contains supports of all fuzzy variables corresponding to the terms placed in the lists "*presence*" and "*decisive character*". We first define three atomic expressions in $A$, i.e., "*the leftmost*" = "*seldom*", "*in the middle*" = "*moderately*" and "*the rightmost*" = "*often*". We thus propose the following constrains for "*the leftmost*" and "*the rightmost*" variables, provided that the abbreviation "*se*" points at the parameters of "*seldom*" [49]:

$$y = \mu_{\text{"seldom"}}(x) = \begin{cases} 1 & \text{for } x \le \alpha_{se}, \\ \dfrac{2(\beta_{se} - \alpha_{se})^2 - (x - \alpha_{se})^2}{2(\beta_{se} - \alpha_{se})^2} & \text{for } \alpha_{se} < x \le \beta_{se}, \\ \dfrac{(\gamma_{se} - x)^2}{2(\gamma_{se} - \beta_{se})^2} & \text{for } \beta_{se} < x < \gamma_{se}, \\ 0 & \text{for } x \ge \gamma_{se}, \end{cases} \tag{3.13}$$

while "*often*" is dependent on the parameters of "*seldom*" in the way

$$y = \mu_{\text{"often"}}(x) =$$
$$\begin{cases} 0 & \text{for } x \le A_l - \gamma_{se}, \\ \dfrac{(x - (A_l - \gamma_{se}))^2}{2((A_l - \beta_{se}) - (A_l - \gamma_{se}))^2} & \text{for } A_l - \gamma_{se} < x \le A_l - \beta_{se}, \\ \dfrac{2((A_l - \alpha_{se}) - (A_l - \beta_{se}))^2 - (x - (A_l - \alpha_{se}))^2}{2((A_l - \alpha_{se}) - (A_l - \beta_{se}))^2} & \text{for } A_l - \beta_{se} < x < A_l - \alpha_{se}, \\ 1 & \text{for } x \ge A_l - \alpha_{se}. \end{cases} \tag{3.14}$$

After transforming Eq. (3.13) we realize that it is identical with $\mu_{\text{"seldom"}}(x) = 1 - s(x, \alpha_{se}, \beta_{se}, \gamma_{se})$ while Eq. (3.14) is identified with $\mu_{\text{"often"}}(x) = s(x, \alpha_{of}, \beta_{of}, \gamma_{of})$, where $\alpha_{of} = A_l - \gamma_{se}$, $\beta_{of} = A_l - \beta_{se}$, $\gamma_{of} = A_l - \alpha_{se}$, and the abbreviation "*of*" is intended for the variable "*often*". Let us also suppose that $\gamma_{se} = \alpha_{of} = \dfrac{A_l}{2}$.

**Example 3.9**

We accept as a common range for all the variables the reference set $A$ = [0, 1, 2, …, 100] by following the results obtained in Ex. 2.15. Then $A_l$ takes the value of 100 as the largest value in the range $A$. If we also state the values of $\alpha_{se}$, $\beta_{se}$, $\gamma_{se}$ as 30, 40, 50, respectively, in "*seldom*" and "*often*" we then will implement the membership functions of the "*leftmost*" and "*rightmost*" atomic words derived as the split definitions

$$y = \mu_{\text{"}seldom\text{"}}(x) = \begin{cases} 1 & \text{for} \quad x \le 30, \\ \dfrac{2(40-30)^2 - (x-30)^2}{2(40-30)^2} & \text{for} \quad 30 < x \le 40, \\ \dfrac{(x-50)^2}{2(50-40)^2} & \text{for} \quad 40 < x < 50, \\ 0 & \text{for} \quad x \ge 50, \end{cases} \tag{3.15}$$

and

$$y = \mu_{\text{"}often\text{"}}(x) =$$
$$\begin{cases} 0 & \text{for } x \le 100-50, \\ \dfrac{(x-(100-50))^2}{2((100-40)-(100-50))^2} & \text{for } 100-50 < x \le 100-40, \\ \dfrac{2((100-30)-(100-40))^2 - (x-(100-30))^2}{2((100-30)-(100-40))^2} & \text{for } 100-40 < x < 100-30, \\ 1 & \text{for } x \ge 100-30. \end{cases} \tag{3.16}$$

We emphasize that we only need to define "*the leftmost*" description to implement both membership functions for "*seldom*" and "*often*".

The membership function of "*moderately*" still remains equal to the function introduced by (2.6), and is adopted here as an atomic expression formulated as "*in the middle*". This takes a form of

$$\pi\left(x, \frac{A_l}{2} - \alpha_{se}, \frac{A_l}{2}\right) = \begin{cases} s\left(x, \alpha_{se}, \dfrac{A_l + 2\alpha_{se}}{4}, \dfrac{A_l}{2}\right) & \text{for} \quad x \le \dfrac{A_l}{2}, \\ 1 - s\left(x, \dfrac{A_l}{2}, \dfrac{3A_l - 2\alpha_{se}}{4}, A_l - \alpha_{se}\right) & \text{for} \quad \text{x} > \dfrac{A_l}{2}. \end{cases} \tag{3.17}$$

**Example 3.10**

For $A_l = 100$ and $\alpha_{se} = 30$, which generate the borders in (3.17), the last formula becomes

$$y = \pi(x,20,50) = \begin{cases} s(x,30,40,50) & \text{for} \quad x \le 50, \\ 1 - s(x,50,60,70) & \text{for} \quad x > 50. \end{cases}$$

We often need to widen the list of expressions coming into existence from the atomic words with the membership functions established in Ex. 3.9. If we want to use the descriptions "*very seldom*" or "*rather seldom*", then we should adjust the membership functions of new fuzzy variables that possess names consisting of both the atomic words and hedges. The hedges are interpreted as additional descriptions (usually adjectives) added to atomic words. In the word compositions "*very seldom*" or "*rather seldom*", the hedges are found as "*very*" and "*rather*". To generate membership functions of sophisticated linguistic formulations, including such adjectives as "*very*", "*rather*", "*almost*" and the like, we add a parameter $\delta$ to the parameters $\alpha_{se}$, $\beta_{se}$, $\gamma_{se}$, already existing in (3.13) and (3.14). The action of the parameter $\delta$ introduces either a narrowing or a widening effect in membership functions of these fuzzy variables that are derived from atomic expressions.

**Example 3.11**

We suggest the formulas of membership functions with hedges for two groups of fuzzy variables. We modify Eq. (3.15) as

$$y = \mu_{\text{"}hedge\ seldom\text{"}}(x) = \begin{cases} 1 & \text{for } x \le 30\delta, \\ \dfrac{2\delta^2(40-30)^2 - (x-30\delta)^2}{2\delta^2(40-30)^2} & \text{for } 30\delta < x \le 40\delta, \\ \dfrac{(x-50\delta)^2}{2\delta^2(50-40)^2} & \text{for } 40\delta < x < 50\delta, \\ 0 & \text{for } x \ge 50\delta, \end{cases} \tag{3.18}$$

to produce membership functions of the variables originating from "*seldom*".

The changes in (3.16) made as

$$y = \mu_{\text{"}hedge\ often\text{"}}(x) =$$
$$\begin{cases} 0 & \text{for } x \le 100 - 50\delta, \\ \dfrac{(x-(100-50\delta))^2}{2\delta^2((100-40)-(100-50))^2} & \text{for } 100-50\delta < x \le 100-40\delta, \\ \dfrac{2\delta^2((100-30)-(100-40))^2-(x-(100-30\delta))^2}{2\delta^2((100-30)-(100-40))^2} & \text{for } 100-40\delta < x < 100-30\delta, \\ 1 & \text{for } x \le 100-30\delta, \end{cases} \tag{3.19}$$

give a class of functions possessing "*often*" in their names.

The parameter $\delta$ works in accordance with the following criteria [49]:

1. $\delta = 1$ where no hedge in (3.18) and (3.19) is needed (*empty hedge*);
2. $0 < \delta < 1$ is applied for hedges with narrowing effects;
3. $\delta > 1$ is introduced for hedges with widening effects.

**Example 3.12**

We have tested different values of a parameter $\delta$ to finally decide that the most appropriate values of $\delta$ in the case of "*seldom*" can be stated as $\delta = 0.75$ for "*very seldom*", $\delta = 0.5$ for "*very, very seldom*" = "*almost never*", $\delta = 0.25$ for "*very, very, very seldom*" = "*never*" and $\delta = 1.25$ for "*rather seldom*". The values of $\delta <$ 1 will narrow supports of "*hedge seldom*" variables but $\delta > 1$, on the contrary, widens an outlook of "*rather seldom*".

The graphs of the membership functions generated by "*seldom*" when taking into account the parameters designed above are depicted in Fig. 3.4.

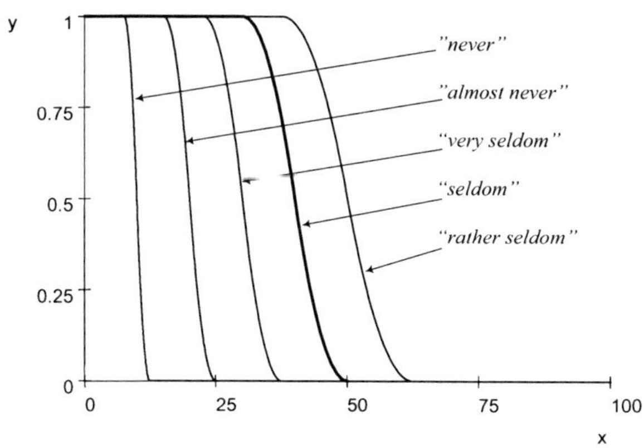


Figure 3.4: The membership functions of fuzzy variables generated by "*seldom*"

The formula (3.19) yields further composed structures proceeding from the other atomic word "*often*". By determining $\delta = 0.75$ we generate the membership function of "*very often*", $\delta = 0.5$ gives "*very, very often*" = "*almost always*" and we get "*very, very, very often*" = "*always*" for $\delta = 0.25$. To create the membership function of "*rather often*" we exploit the widening effect of $\delta$ and decide its value as $\delta = 1.25$.

The common result of employing the parameter $\delta$ as a factor changing the membership function of "*often*" for the sophisticated expressions containing this word is seen in Fig. 3.5.

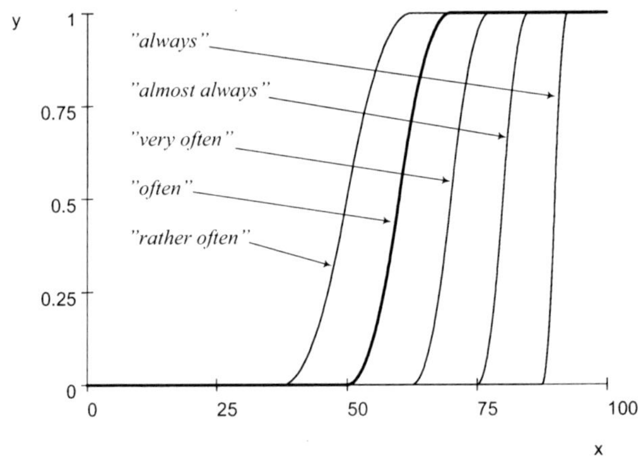


Figure 3.5: The membership functions of fuzzy variables generated by "*often*"

We now sample the results of all latest investigations that have led to the construction of new membership functions. These, as fuzzy variables shown in Fig. 3.6, represent the terms of "*presence*" and "*decisive character*".

In the further step of our efforts leading to a creation of the *SD* matrix, we desire to extract only one value of the support that represents each fuzzy variable belonging to "*presence*" and "*decisive character*". It seems to be reliable to accept, as a representative, this element of the variable support that is treated as a certain border of the variable's membership function. We can establish the boundary value, *x*, as the *x*-coordinate of an intersection point between the line $\mu_{variable}(x) = 1$ and a part of the membership function in which $\mu_{variable}(x) < 1$. The expressions coming from "*seldom*" have thus the borders determined as $x = 30\delta$ while the descriptions created by "*often*" form the group with representatives equal to $x = (A_l = 100) - 30\delta$.

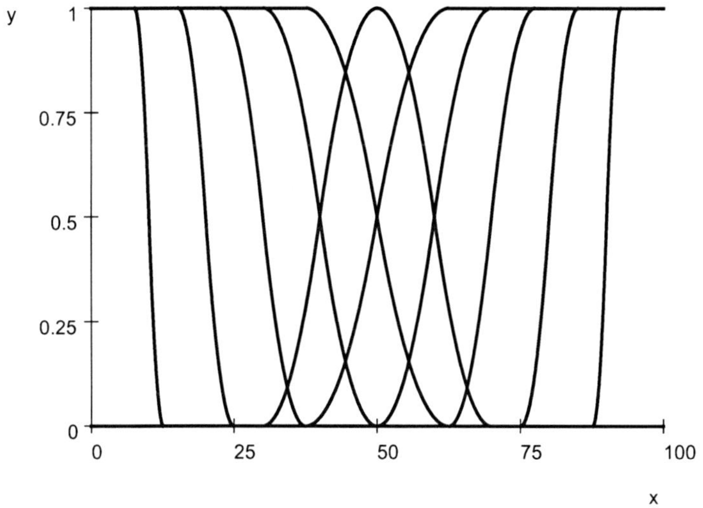


Figure 3.6: The terms from the lists "*presence*" and "*decisive character*"

**Example 3.13**

The representatives of the variables "*never*",..., "*always*" are sampled in Table 3.1.

Table 3.1: The representatives of the variables "*never*", ..., "*always*"

| Fuzzy variables | $\delta$ | The representatives for the fuzzy variables in the reference set [0, 100] |
|---|---|---|
| "*never*" | 0.25 | $x = 30 \cdot 0.25 = 7.5$ |
| "*almost never*" | 0.5 | $x = 30 \cdot 0.5 = 15$ |
| "*very seldom*" | 0.75 | $x = 30 \cdot 0.75 = 22.5$ |
| "*seldom*" | 1 | $x = 30 \cdot 1 = 30$ |
| "*rather seldom*" | 1.25 | $x = 30 \cdot 1.25 = 37.5$ |
| "*moderately*" | – | $x = 50$ |
| "*rather often*" | 1.25 | $x = 100 - 30 \cdot 1.25 = 62.5$ |
| "*often*" | 1 | $x = 100 - 30 \cdot 1 = 70$ |
| "*very often*" | 0.75 | $x = 100 - 30 \cdot 0.75 = 77.5$ |
| "*almost always*" | 0.5 | $x = 100 - 30 \cdot 0.5 = 85$ |
| "*always*" | 0.25 | $x = 100 - 30 \cdot 0.25 = 92.5$ |

To give expression to the verbal descriptions of presence and decisive character via values of the membership degrees, we finally plan a common restriction

$$\mu_{"common"}(x) = s(x, \alpha_{common}, \beta_{common}, \gamma_{common}) \tag{3.20}$$

that completely covers the space formed for the representative values from Table 3.1.

**Example 3.14**

Let us accept $\alpha_{common}$ = 7.5, $\beta_{common}$ = 50 and $\gamma_{common}$ = 92.5 in (3.20). It should be mentioned that the borders of the space for "*common*" are decided to be equal to 7.5 respectively 92.5 to obtain the value of zero as the membership degree standing for "*never*", and the value of one assigned to "*always*" in accordance with the physicians' ability to interpret "*never*" and "*always*". By setting the numbers from the last column of Table 3.1 in (3.20) as $x$-values, we decide the association between the names of variables and the corresponding membership degrees assigned to them. We state the results of appropriate computations in Table 3.2.

Table 3.2: The numerical description of fuzzy variables in "*presence*"

| Fuzzy variables | $x$ | $\mu_{"common"}(x)$ |
|---|---|---|
| "*never*" | 7.5 | 0 |
| "*almost never*" | 15 | 0.016 |
| "*very seldom*" | 22.5 | 0.062 |
| "*seldom*" | 30 | 0.14 |
| "*rather seldom*" | 37.5 | 0.25 |
| "*moderately*" | 50 | 0.5 |
| "*rather often*" | 62.5 | 0.75 |
| "*often*" | 70 | 0.86 |
| "*very often*" | 77.5 | 0.938 |
| "*almost always*" | 85 | 0.984 |
| "*always*" | 92.5 | 1 |

Table 3.2 provides us with the information on how to tie the words taking place in the lists, "*presence*" and "*decisive character*", to real numbers that replace them in the fuzzy relations "*symptom – diagnosis*", which we will generate in the next subsection.

### 3.4.2 Relations of "*Presence*" and "*Decisive Character*"

When a physician is asked to decide, e.g., the presence of a symptom in the corresponding diagnosis, then he should only choose a word from the list containing the items that determine "*presence*". In computations assisting a mathematical model a number replaces the verbal expression approved by the physician.

**Example 3.15**

We consider three diagnoses $D_1$ = "*high risk of cardiovascular diseases*", $D_2$ = "*coronary heart disease*" and $D_3$ = "*myocardial infarct*". These are associated with the symptoms $S_1$, …, $S_{10}$ already discussed in Ex. 3.1. To answer the questions: "*How often is $S_j$ found in $D_k$?*" and "*How often is $S_j$ decisive for $D_k$?*", $j = 1, \ldots, 10$, $k = 1, 2, 3$, the physician selects a word from the list defining "*presence*" and "*decisive character*". His answers are collected in Table 3.3.

This table inserts the information in the mathematical model of diagnosing sometimes called "medical knowledge" because of its expressing a correlation between clinical symptoms and diagnoses. The relations *PS*, made for individual patients vary a lot from each other, but "the medical knowledge" remains invariant when looking for the most reliable diagnosis with regards to the same symptoms.

Table 3.3: Linguistic frequency and importance of $S_1$, …, $S_{10}$ in $D_1$, $D_2$, $D_3$

| Symptoms | Presence | | | Decisive character | | |
|---|---|---|---|---|---|---|
| | $D_1$ | $D_2$ | $D_3$ | $D_1$ | $D_2$ | $D_3$ |
| $S_1$ | *often* | *often* | *often* | *often* | *often* | *almost always* |
| $S_2$ | *almost never* | *rather seldom* | *very often* | *very seldom* | *moderately* | *often* |
| $S_3$ | *rather often* | *often* | *often* | *almost always* | *often* | *often* |
| $S_4$ | *often* | *very often* | *very often* | *often* | *often* | *often* |
| $S_5$ | *almost never* | *often* | *very often* | *almost never* | *almost always* | *always* |
| $S_6$ | *almost never* | *seldom* | *rather often* | *almost never* | *seldom* | *often* |
| $S_7$ | *almost never* | *very seldom* | *moderately* | *almost never* | *seldom* | *very often* |
| $S_8$ | *very often* | *often* | *often* | *very often* | *often* | *often* |
| $S_9$ | *very often* | *very often* | *very often* | *very often* | *very often* | *often* |
| $S_{10}$ | *often* | *rather often* | *rather often* | *often* | *often* | *moderately* |

The results obtained in Table 3.2 are used to the expressions put in Table 3.3 to replace them by numbers shown in Table 3.4.

For example, we ask a physician about the association of symptom $S_{10}$ = "*obesity*" and diagnosis $D_3$ = "*myocardial infarct*" in the context of "*presence*". As an answer we get a piece of information stated as "*rather often*". By applying Eq. (3.20) we have computed $\mu_{\text{"}common\text{"}}(62.5) = 1 - 2\left(\dfrac{62.5 - 92.5}{92.5 - 7.5}\right)^2 \approx 0.75$. It means that the physician's statement will be utilized as 0.75 in a mathematical diagnostic model.

Table 3.4: Numerical frequency and importance of $S_1, \ldots, S_{10}$ in $D_1, D_2, D_3$

| Symptoms | Presence | | | Decisive character | | |
|---|---|---|---|---|---|---|
| | $D_1$ | $D_2$ | $D_3$ | $D_1$ | $D_2$ | $D_3$ |
| $S_1$ | 0.86 | 0.86 | 0.86 | 0.86 | 0.86 | 0.984 |
| $S_2$ | 0.016 | 0.25 | 0.938 | 0.062 | 0.5 | 0.86 |
| $S_3$ | 0.75 | 0.86 | 0.86 | 0.984 | 0.86 | 0.86 |
| $S_4$ | 0.86 | 0.938 | 0.938 | 0.86 | 0.86 | 0.86 |
| $S_5$ | 0.016 | 0.86 | 0.938 | 0.016 | 0.984 | 1 |
| $S_6$ | 0.016 | 0.14 | 0.75 | 0.016 | 0.14 | 0.86 |
| $S_7$ | 0.016 | 0.062 | 0.5 | 0.016 | 0.14 | 0.938 |
| $S_8$ | 0.938 | 0.86 | 0.86 | 0.938 | 0.86 | 0.86 |
| $S_9$ | 0,938 | 0.938 | 0.938 | 0.938 | 0.938 | 0.86 |
| $S_{10}$ | 0.86 | 0.75 | 0.75 | 0.86 | 0.86 | 0.5 |

The contents of Table 3.4 can be rewritten as two matrices named "*symptom – presence*" and "*symptom – decisive character*". The first matrix forms a fuzzy relation $SD_P$ that informs us about the presence of symptoms in the considered diagnoses. The other matrix creates a relation $SD_D$ containing the knowledge about importance of the symptoms for the diagnoses. We introduce the relations as the matrices

$$SD_P = \begin{array}{c} \\ S_1 \\ S_2 \\ S_3 \\ S_4 \\ S_5 \\ S_6 \\ S_7 \\ S_8 \\ S_9 \\ S_{10} \end{array} \begin{array}{c} \begin{array}{ccc} D_1 & D_2 & D_3 \end{array} \\ \begin{bmatrix} 0.86 & 0.86 & 0.86 \\ 0.016 & 0.25 & 0.938 \\ 0.75 & 0.86 & 0.86 \\ 0.86 & 0.938 & 0.938 \\ 0.016 & 0.86 & 0.938 \\ 0.016 & 0.14 & 0.75 \\ 0.016 & 0.062 & 0.5 \\ 0.938 & 0.86 & 0.86 \\ 0.938 & 0.938 & 0.938 \\ 0.86 & 0.75 & 0.75 \end{bmatrix} \end{array} \qquad SD_D = \begin{array}{c} \\ S_1 \\ S_2 \\ S_3 \\ S_4 \\ S_5 \\ S_6 \\ S_7 \\ S_8 \\ S_9 \\ S_{10} \end{array} \begin{array}{c} \begin{array}{ccc} D_1 & D_2 & D_3 \end{array} \\ \begin{bmatrix} 0.86 & 0.86 & 0.984 \\ 0.062 & 0.5 & 0.86 \\ 0.984 & 0.86 & 0.86 \\ 0.86 & 0.86 & 0.86 \\ 0.016 & 0.984 & 1 \\ 0.016 & 0.14 & 0.86 \\ 0.016 & 0.14 & 0.938 \\ 0.938 & 0.86 & 0.86 \\ 0.938 & 0.938 & 0.86 \\ 0.86 & 0.86 & 0.5 \end{bmatrix} \end{array}.$$

The relations: $PS$ discussed in Section 3.3, $SD_P$ and $SD_D$ constitute important components in the set of equations being the mathematical formalizations of the compositional rule of inference *modus ponens*, already mentioned in Section 3.2. Even another mathematical law, *modus tollens*, is utilized to improve the decision making process regarding the most reliable choice of a diagnosis based on clinical symptoms.

## 3.5 The *Patient – Diagnosis* Relation

Fuzzy relations $PS$, $SD_P$ and $SD_D$ are elements of fuzzy relation equations that bring solutions regarded as fuzzy relations of the type $PD$ = "*patient – diagnosis*". These new relations contain pairs ($P_1$, $D_k$), $k$ = 1, 2,..., $p$. By superposing the fuzzy relations in the way suggested in Eq. (2.21), we obtain equations with the operation of max-min type.

We return to Def. 3.1, which develops the meaning of the compositional rule of inference *modus ponens*, already cited in Subsection 3.2, to recall its diagnostic interpretation:

"If symptom $S_j$ appears in patient $P_1$ with the membership degree $\mu_{PS}(P_1,S_j)$"

and

"If the presence of $S_j$ results in $D_k$ with the membership degree $\mu_{SD_P}(S_j,D_k)$ or $\mu_{SD_D}(S_j,D_k)$"

then

"Diagnosis $D_k$ occurs in patient $P_1$ with the membership degree $\mu_{PD}(P_1, D_k)$".

Fuzzy relations, replacing the statements of the rule formulated above, are components of a fuzzy relation equation [2, 3]

$$PD_1 = PS \circ SD_P, \tag{3.21}$$

in which the relation $PD_1$ has the membership function (2.21) customized as

$$\mu_{PD_1}(P_1,D_k) = \max_{S_j \in S}(\min(\mu_{PS}(P_1,S_j),\mu_{SD_P}(S_j,D_k))) . \tag{3.22}$$

The relation $SD_D$ has found its place in the next relation equation

$$PD_2 = PS \circ SD_D . \tag{3.23}$$

The membership function of $PD_2$ is derived as

$$\mu_{PD_2}(P_1,D_k) = \max_{S_j \in S}(\min(\mu_{PS}(P_1,S_j),\mu_{SD_D}(S_j,D_k))) \tag{3.24}$$

for $j$ = 1, 2, …, $n$, $k$ = 1, 2, …, $p$.

The relations $PD_1$ and $PD_2$, discussed in Eqs (3.21) and (3.23), are involved in an equation

$$PD_3 = \min(PD_1,PD_2) , \tag{3.25}$$

where the membership function of $PD_3$ is constructed as

$$\mu_{PD_3}(P_1, D_k) = \min(\mu_{PD_1}(P_1, D_k), \mu_{PD_2}(P_1, D_k)). \tag{3.26}$$

The relation $PD_3$ decides about an acceptance of the diagnosis in patient $P_1$ by means of comparing the membership degrees in $PD_3$. The higher the membership degree of the diagnosis $D_k$ in $P_1$ is, the more certain the approval of $D_k$ will be.

The membership degrees appearing in the row of $P_1$ in $PD_3$ sometimes do not differ essentially to indicate an optimal diagnosis as a clear-cut decision. They may sometimes differ in minutely; therefore it is also recommended that one analyzes the possibility of rejecting the diagnoses.

Another rule of inference, known as *modus tollens*, is a logical law of the shape

IF "NOT $q$" AND "$p$ IMPLIES $q$" THEN "NOT $p$".

If we interpret the premises of the law as

"NOT $q$" = "Symptom $S_j$ does not appear in patient $P_1$ with the membership degree $1 - \mu_{PS}(P_1, S_j)$"

and

"$p$ IMPLIES $q$" = "$D_k$ requires the presence of $S_j$ with the membership degree $\mu_{SD_P}(S_j, D_k)$"

then we draw the conclusion

"NOT $p$" = "Diagnosis $D_k$ is rejected in patient $P_1$ with the membership degree $\mu_{PD}(P_1, D_k)$".

We interpret the mathematical meaning of the *modus tollens* law as an equation

$$PD_4 = (1 - PS) \circ SD_P \cdot \tag{3.27}$$

The membership function of $PD_4$ is presented in the form of

$$\mu_{PD_4}(P_1, D_k) = \max_{S_j \in S}(\min(1 - \mu_{PS}(P_1, S_j), \mu_{SD_P}(S_j, D_k))), \tag{3.28}$$

for each diagnosis from the set $D$.

By applying the *double negation* law "NOT(NOT $q$)) = $q$" we modify *modus tollens* as a statement

IF "$q$" AND "$p$ IMPLIES (NOT $q$)" THEN "NOT $p$."

A translation of the premises in the last version of the *modus tollens* law into an understandable medical sentence can be formulated as follows.

If

"$q$" = "Symptom $S_j$ appears in patient $P_1$ with the degree $\mu_{PS}(P_1, S_j)$"

and
"$q$ IMPLIES (NOT $p$)" = "$D_k$ does not need the presence of $S_j$ with the membership degree $1-\mu_{SD_P}(S_j,D_k)$"
then we will come to the thesis
"NOT $p$" = "Diagnosis $D_k$ is rejected for patient $P_1$ with the membership degree $\mu_{PD}(P_1, D_k)$".

The last adaptation of *modus tollens* has given rise to a fuzzy relation involved in the diagnostic process in the way of a composition

$$PD_5 = PS \circ (1 - SD_P), \tag{3.29}$$

where the relation $PD_5$ is characterized by the membership function

$$\mu_{PD_5}(P_1,D_k) = \max_{S_j \in S}(\min(\mu_{PS}(P_1,S_j),1-\mu_{SD_P}(S_j,D_k))) . \tag{3.30}$$

The fuzzy relations $PD_4$ and $PD_5$ resolve of the rejection of a diagnosis assisting patient $P_1$. The higher the value of the membership degree associated with the diagnosis in $PD_4$ and $PD_5$ is, the greater the certainty of the diagnosis rejection will be.

The formulas (3.22), (3.24), (3.26), (3.28) and (3.30) are valid for $j = 1, 2,\ldots, n$ and $k = 1, 2,\ldots, p$.

The final decision concerning the acceptance of a proper diagnosis assumes the simultaneous and thorough comparison of the membership degrees originating from the relations $PD_3$, $PD_4$ and $PD_5$.

**Example 3.16**

We can already provide patient $P_1$ with the relations $PS$, $SD_P$ and $SD_D$ that have been determined for his sake in Ex. 3.8 and 3.15 respectively. A computing process of the relations $PD_1$–$PD_5$ is carried through by involving Eqs (3.21)–(3.30), in turn, as it is executed below.

00

If

$$PS = P_1\begin{bmatrix} \overset{S_1}{1} & \overset{S_2}{0.515} & \overset{S_3}{0.913} & \overset{S_4}{0.653} & \overset{S_5}{0.345} & \overset{S_6}{0.632} & \overset{S_7}{0.720} & \overset{S_8}{0.9} & \overset{S_9}{0.0004} & \overset{S_{10}}{0.353} \end{bmatrix}$$

then we would like to have access to the relation $SD_P$ as the second component in Eq. (3.21) to appreciate $PD_1$.

Hence,

$$PD_1 = PS \circ SD_P$$

or

$$PD_1 = P_1 \overset{\begin{array}{cccccccccc} S_1 & S_2 & S_3 & S_4 & S_5 & S_6 & S_7 & S_8 & S_9 & S_{10} \end{array}}{[\begin{array}{cccccccccc} 1 & 0.515 & 0.913 & 0.653 & 0.345 & 0.632 & 0.720 & 0.9 & 0.0004 & 0.353 \end{array}]} \circ$$

$$\begin{array}{c} \\ S_1 \\ S_2 \\ S_3 \\ S_4 \\ S_5 \\ S_6 \\ S_7 \\ S_8 \\ S_9 \\ S_{10} \end{array} \begin{array}{c} \begin{array}{ccc} D_1 & D_2 & D_3 \end{array} \\ \begin{bmatrix} 0.86 & 0.86 & 0.86 \\ 0.016 & 0.25 & 0.938 \\ 0.75 & 0.86 & 0.86 \\ 0.86 & 0.938 & 0.938 \\ 0.016 & 0.86 & 0.938 \\ 0.016 & 0.14 & 0.75 \\ 0.016 & 0.062 & 0.5 \\ 0.938 & 0.86 & 0.86 \\ 0.938 & 0.938 & 0.938 \\ 0.86 & 0.75 & 0.75 \end{bmatrix} \end{array} = P_1 \overset{\begin{array}{ccc} D_1 & D_2 & D_3 \end{array}}{[0.9 \quad 0.86 \quad 0.86]}.$$

To calculate a membership degree for the pair ($P_1$, $D_1$) we follow the operations recommended by (3.22). Hence, $\mu_{PD_1}(P_1, D_1)$ = max(min(1, 0.86), min(0.515, 0.016), min(0.913, 0.75), min(0.653, 0.86), min(0.345, 0.016), min(0.632, 0.016), min(0.720, 0.016), min(0.9, 0.938), min(0.0004, 0.938), min(0.353, 0.86)) = max(0.86, 0.016, 0.75, 0.653, 0.016, 0.016, 0.016, 0.9, 0.0004, 0.353) = 0.9.

In accordance with (3.23) and (3.24) we evaluate

$$PD_2 = PS \circ SD_D = P_1 \overset{\begin{array}{ccc} D_1 & D_2 & D_3 \end{array}}{[0.913 \quad 0.86 \quad 0.984]}$$

and by returning to (3.25) and (3.26), we obtain

$$PD_3 = \min(PD_1, PD_2) = P_1 \overset{\begin{array}{ccc} D_1 & D_2 & D_3 \end{array}}{[0.9 \quad 0.86 \quad 0.86]}$$

as the final decision of accepting the diagnosis.

Since the membership degrees in $PD_3$ are almost equal, we should examine the possibility of rejecting the diagnoses as a supplementary decisive factor. In further computations we exploit two complements to matrices already introduced. Let us consequently find 1 – $PS$ as a table

$$1 - PS = P_1 \overset{\begin{array}{cccccccccc} S_1 & S_2 & S_3 & S_4 & S_5 & S_6 & S_7 & S_8 & S_9 & S_{10} \end{array}}{[\begin{array}{cccccccccc} 0 & 0.485 & 0.087 & 0.347 & 0.655 & 0.368 & 0.280 & 0.1 & 0.9996 & 0.647 \end{array}]}$$

filled with membership degrees that are calculated by subtracting $\mu_{PS}(P_1, D_k)$ from one, $k = 1, \ldots, p$. The other matrix $1 - SD_P$, is an algebraic complement to one and has a form

$$1 - SD_P = \begin{array}{c} \\ S_1 \\ S_2 \\ S_3 \\ S_4 \\ S_5 \\ S_6 \\ S_7 \\ S_8 \\ S_9 \\ S_{10} \end{array} \begin{array}{c} \begin{array}{ccc} D_1 & D_2 & D_3 \end{array} \\ \begin{bmatrix} 0.14 & 0.14 & 0.14 \\ 0.984 & 0.75 & 0.062 \\ 0.25 & 0.14 & 0.14 \\ 0.14 & 0.062 & 0.062 \\ 0.984 & 0.14 & 0.062 \\ 0.984 & 0.86 & 0.25 \\ 0.984 & 0.938 & 0.5 \\ 0.062 & 0.14 & 0.14 \\ 0.062 & 0.062 & 0.062 \\ 0.14 & 0.25 & 0.25 \end{bmatrix} \end{array}.$$

We now use (3.27) and (3.28) to state the contents of $PD_4$ as the table

$$PD_4 = (1 - PS) \circ SD_P = P_1 \overset{\begin{array}{ccc} D_1 & D_2 & D_3 \end{array}}{\begin{bmatrix} 0.938 & 0.938 & 0.938 \end{bmatrix}}.$$

$PD_4$ is the first matrix that provides us with a decision about excluding the diagnoses. By adopting (3.29) and (3.30) we calculate the entries of the matrix $PD_5$ that closes the series of matrices participating in the decision making process with respect to the optimal diagnosis. $PD_5$, which is founded on the complement of the fuzzy relation $SD_P$, possesses the following membership degrees

$$PD_5 = PS \circ (1 - SD_P) = P_1 \overset{\begin{array}{ccc} D_1 & D_2 & D_3 \end{array}}{\begin{bmatrix} 0.720 & 0.720 & 0.500 \end{bmatrix}}.$$

To make the final decision let us sum up the obtained data in Table 3.5

Table 3.5: $P_1$'s diagnostic decision based on $PD_3$, $PD_4$ and $PD_5$

| | $PD_3$ | | | $PD_4$ | | | $PD_5$ | | | Decision |
|---|---|---|---|---|---|---|---|---|---|---|
| Patient | $D_1$ | $D_2$ | $D_3$ | $D_1$ | $D_2$ | $D_3$ | $D_1$ | $D_2$ | $D_3$ | |
| $P_1$ | 0.90 | 0.86 | 0.86 | 0.938 | 0.938 | 0.938 | 0.72 | 0.72 | 0.5 | $D_1$ or $D_3$ |

After carrying out a thorough analysis of all membership degrees, we agree with the decision of accepting $D_1$ or $D_3$ as the disease that patient $P_1$ suffers from.

Unfortunately, we cannot decide which disease is right since the obtained information is not clear. We motivate making our choice in the way described below:

1. The membership degree of $D_1$ in $PD_3$ is the largest value that convinces us to approve $D_1$ as the most plausible disease;
2. The matrix $PD_4$ has all the membership degrees equal, which means that the decision is lacking;
3. Finally, by rejecting the diagnoses $D_1$ and $D_2$ in $P_1$, since they have the highest membership degrees in $PD_5$, we leave $D_3$ as the most probable diagnosis in the considered patient.

The physician has sampled the data about the patient's state and confirmed that $P_1$'s health state is very severe. He risks a myocardial infarct in the substantial grade, which justifies our doubtful decision between $D_1$ and $D_3$.

Let us also provide a bit of information concerning another patient $P_2$.

**Example 3.17**

The data sample for $P_2$ is placed in the matrix $PS$ in the symptom order as

$$\begin{array}{rcccccccccc} & S_1 & S_2 & S_3 & S_4 & S_5 & S_6 & S_7 & S_8 & S_9 & S_{10} \\ PS = P_2[ & 0 & 0.2 & 0.4 & 0.5 & 0.1 & 0.3 & 0.8 & 0.9 & 0.8 & 0.6\ ]. \end{array}$$

Table 3.6 contains membership degrees that describe $P_2$'s diagnostic conditions to decide his most credible diagnosis.

Table 3.6: $P_2$'s diagnostic decision based on $PD_3$, $PD_4$ and $PD_5$

| Patient | $PD_3$ | | | $PD_4$ | | | $PD_5$ | | | Decision |
|---|---|---|---|---|---|---|---|---|---|---|
| | $D_1$ | $D_2$ | $D_3$ | $D_1$ | $D_2$ | $D_3$ | $D_1$ | $D_2$ | $D_3$ | |
| $P_1$ | 0.90 | 0.86 | 0.86 | 0.86 | 0.86 | 0.9 | 0.8 | 0.8 | 0.5 | $D_3$ |

Once again we meet the patient's case that is not easy to diagnose. The differences among the membership degrees representing $PD_3$ are not substantial enough to indicate the diagnosis accepted for the patient. Even the degrees in the rejection matrix $PD_4$, as close to each other, do not convince us completely about the choice of a proper diagnosis assigned to $P_2$. Only the informative character of $PD_5$ can be considered as reliable because of essential differences among the membership degrees placed in this relation. Since the value of $D_3$ is smallest of all in $PD_5$ then we will admit that the recognized diagnosis is identified as $D_3$. The patient's medical reports certify this choice as well.

We can observe some harmful effects of the maximum and minimum operations included in compositions of relations. These operations deprive many membership degrees of their power in the final decisions. Therefore we need to use "softer" calculations that take into considerations all values presented by the matrices "*patient – symptom*" and "*symptom – diagnosis*".

Many patient cases that do not deliver diagnostic specifications in order to make a clear choice among diagnoses should be supported by complementary solutions. We intend to discuss the supplementary details of diagnostic models in the next part of the dissertation.

# 4 Complementary Solutions in Diagnostic Models

## 4.1 Introduction

We should admit that the case of patient $P_1$ in Ex. 3.16 has not been very easy to solve especially when you consider the proper interpretation of $PD_3$. By equipping us with equal values of the membership degrees it has not made it easy enough to make the proper choice of an unknown diagnosis.

Moreover, the patient has been examined only once according to existing reports about his health. If the patient visits the doctor's office more than one time, then we can notice some changes in values of biological parameters under consideration. The increasing or decreasing values of clinical symptoms, when observing them many times, can absolutely exclude this diagnosis that has been approved after the first examination. The analysis of a diagnostic model extended in time could provide us with more accurate information that assists in making a better choice of a disease.

To limit some doubtful diagnostic decisions made by means of mathematical tools, we propose the supplementary solutions handled in this chapter.

## 4.2 OWA Operators in Decision Relations

The results from Ex. 3.16, obtained as the membership degrees taking place in five decision matrices, are possible to interpret even if the values in $PD_3$ have become equal or the values in $PD_4$ have not varied much from each other. Nevertheless, we desire to obtain clearer information that is accessible in the model's final relations and to be capable of conveying a right conclusion.

The almost equal membership degrees calculated on account of (3.22), (3.24), (3.26), (3.28) and (3.30) have been influenced by an action of the maximum operation. By taking the maximum values in the sets of minimum compounds consisting of $\mu_{PS}$ and $\mu_{SD}$ we have lost a large part of the useful information since only the largest values of compounds have affected output data. Even the application of (2.23) or (2.24) does not eliminate an unfavourable impact of the maximum operator.

To prevent a loss of valuable explanations in the future let us suggest another concatenation operation in a composition of two matrices, i.e., such a one which takes into consideration all membership degrees included in $PS$ and $SD$.

Elisabeth Rakus-Andersson: *Fuzzy and Rough Techniques in Medical Diagnosis and Medication*, StudFuzz **212**, 63–91 (2007)
www.springerlink.com 

A new definition considering weights is now proven to make diagnostic results clearly interpretable. To accomplish new computations that should lead to an easier analysis of final results in the diagnostic model, we suggest making an acquaintance with OWA aggregating operations. We thus cite a general definition of an OWA operator [46, 82, 84, 86].

**Definition 4.1**

If $x_1$, $x_2$, …, $x_n$ are some estimates of the same quantity $x$, then an aggregation operation called Ordered Weighted Averaging (OWA) has a type

$$f(x_1, x_2, ..., x_n) = a_0 + a_1 \cdot x_{(1)} + a_2 \cdot x_{(2)} + \cdots + a_n \cdot x_{(n)}, \qquad (4.1)$$

where $a_0$, $a_1$, …, $a_n$ are constants.

The values $x_{(1)}$, $x_{(2)}$, …, $x_{(n)}$ are described in the terms of minimum and maximum as

- $x_{(1)} = \min(x_1, x_2, ..., x_n)$
- $x_{(2)} = \max(x(1), ..., x(n))$, where $x(i)$ is the minimum of all the values except the $i^{\text{th}}$, i.e.,
  - $x(1) = \min(x_2, x_3, x_4, ..., x_n)$,
  - $x(2) = \min(x_1, x_3, x_4, ..., x_n)$,
  - …
  - $x(n) = \min(x_1, x_2, x_3, ..., x_{n-1})$;
- $x_{(3)} = \max(x(1,2), x(1,3), ..., x(n-1, n))$, where $x(i, j)$ is the minimum of all the values except the $i^{\text{th}}$ and the $j^{\text{th}}$;
- etc.

**Example 4.1**

The mean $\frac{x_1 + x_2}{2}$ is the OWA operation for $a_0 = 0$, $a_1 = a_2 = \frac{1}{2}$. It can be expanded in the series (4.1) as $\frac{1}{2}\min(x_1, x_2) + \frac{1}{2}\max(\min(x_2), \min(x_1))$. If we set $x_1 = 40$ and $x_2 = 30$ then $\frac{1}{2}\min(40,30) + \frac{1}{2}\max(\min(30), \min(40)) = \frac{30}{2} + \frac{40}{2} = 35$ that is the exact value of the arithmetic mean for 30 and 40.

Both Def. 4.1 and Ex. 4.1 should convince us about the classification of an arithmetic mean as a modern OWA operator.

**Definition 4.2**

We recall the general equation $PD = PS \circ SD$ showed in Section 3.2 that constitutes the most important part in the diagnostic model. We define an operation, denoted symbolically by "$\underset{+}{\circ}$" in order to compose two fuzzy relations $PS$ and $SD$ introduced by (3.1) and (3.2) respectively. The membership function of the relation $PD$ is proposed as

$$\mu_{PD}(P_1,D_k) = \frac{\sum_{j=1}^{n} \mu_{PS}(P_1,S_j)\cdot \mu_{SD}(S_j,D_k)}{\sum_{j=1}^{n} \mu_{SD}(S_j,D_k)} = \frac{\mu_{SD}(S_1,D_k)}{\sum_{j=1}^{n} \mu_{SD}(S_j,D_k)}\cdot \mu_{PS}(P_1,S_1) + \cdots + \frac{\mu_{SD}(S_n,D_k)}{\sum_{j=1}^{n} \mu_{SD}(S_j,D_k)}\cdot \mu_{PS}(P_1,S_n). \tag{4.2}$$

The value of the quotient $\mu_{PD}(P_1, D_k)$ is a number belonging to the interval [0, 1]. To explain it we first notice that $\mu_{PS}(P_1,S_j)\cdot \mu_{SD}(S_j,D_k) \le \mu_{SD}(S_j,D_k)$ since both $\mu_{PS}(P_1,S_j)$ and $\mu_{SD}(S_j,D_k)$ are less than one for all $j$ and $k$, $j = 1, \ldots, n$, $k = 1, \ldots, p$. This causes the value of a product to be less than the values of both factors. We thus conclude that the numerator is less than or equal to the denominator, which guarantees that the entire value of the quotient is a member from [0, 1]; therefore it can be approved as a membership degree of the pair $(P_1, D_k)$.

We also notice that the sum placed in the denominator of the quotient never becomes equal to zero, since almost one of the examined symptoms must express any presence or decisive character for diagnoses included in the designed model. This assumption is very important for truthfulness of the diagnostic model that cannot provide operations on undefined structures.

Let us accommodate (4.2) to the assumptions of (4.1). The value of a sum $\mu_{SD}(S_1,D_k)+\cdots+\mu_{SD}(S_n,D_k)$ and even the quantities $\mu_{SD}(S_j,D_k)$ play roles of invariants for different patients, i.e., they become unchangeable for varying collections of $\mu_{PS}(P_1,S_j)$, $j = 1, \ldots, n$. The mentioned invariants can be reasonably regarded as constants in coefficients

$$a_j = \frac{\mu_{SD}(S_j,D_k)}{\mu_{SD}(S_1,D_k)+\cdots+\mu_{SD}(S_n,D_k)} \tag{4.3}$$

used in the sum (4.1). Further,

$$\mu_{PD}(P_1, D_k) = f(\mu_{PS}(P_1, S_1), \ldots, \mu_{PS}(P_1, S_n)) = a_{j_1}\mu_{PS}(P_1, S_1) + \cdots + a_{j_n}\mu_{PS}(P_1, S_n) \quad (4.4)$$

for $k = 1, \ldots, p$. The order of coefficients $a_{j_1}, \ldots, a_{j_n}$ constitutes a new rearrangement of the sequence $a_1, \ldots, a_n$ made in order to fulfil the assumptions of Def. 4.1. After explaining the meaning of (4.3) and (4.4) we can claim that the proposed operation (4.2) is certified to be assigned to the class of OWA operators.

In the suggested formula (4.2) all membership degrees from the relations *PS* and *SD* are equally valuable for computations. This means that each of the values affects a result. The membership degrees of the $k^{\text{th}}$ column belonging to *SD* act as weights that balance the signification of tested symptoms. To summarize, we come to a conclusion that a proposed value of the membership degree for the pair $(P_1, D_k)$, computed by (4.2), has shown itself to be more intermediary when comparing it to an effect of the sharp value of maximum.

Let us accomplish necessary changes in (3.22), (3.24), (3.26), (3.28) and (3.30) to accommodate them to new circumstances forced by (4.2).

We begin with the composition $PD_1 = PS \underset{+}{\circ} SD_P$ to change its membership function as

$$\mu_{PD_1}(P_1, D_k) = \frac{\sum_{j=1}^{n} \mu_{PS}(P_1, S_j) \cdot \mu_{SD_P}(S_j, D_k)}{\sum_{j=1}^{n} \mu_{SD_P}(S_j, D_k)} \quad (4.5)$$

while the relation $PD_2 = PS \underset{+}{\circ} SD_D$ has a membership function derived by the replacement of the relation $SD_P$ by $SD_D$ in (4.5). This yields a result

$$\mu_{PD_2}(P_1, D_k) = \frac{\sum_{j=1}^{n} \mu_{PS}(P_1, S_j) \cdot \mu_{SD_D}(S_j, D_k)}{\sum_{j=1}^{n} \mu_{SD_D}(S_j, D_k)} \quad (4.6)$$

for $j = 1, 2, \ldots, n$, $k = 1, 2, \ldots, p$.

The relations calculated by applying of (4.5) and (4.6) are involved in the equation $PD_3 = \text{mean}(PD_1, PD_2)$ in which the relation $PD_3$ is characterized by a membership function

$$\mu_{PD_3}(P_1,D_k)=\frac{\mu_{PD_1}(P_1,D_k)+\mu_{PD_2}(P_1,D_k)}{2}. \tag{4.7}$$

The membership degrees of $PD_3$ decide, as before, the approval of the most possible diagnosis in a diagnostic hierarchy.

We upgrade diagnoses in another hierarchical order when we try to reject them. To exclude diagnoses which a patient cannot suffer from, we prepare a membership function of $PD_4=(1-PS)\underset{+}{\circ}SD_P$ as

$$\mu_{PD_4}(P_1,D_k)=\frac{\sum_{j=1}^{n}(1-\mu_{PS}(P_1,S_j))\cdot\mu_{SD_P}(S_j,D_k)}{\sum_{j=1}^{n}\mu_{SD_P}(S_j,D_k)} \tag{4.8}$$

for each diagnosis from the set $D$.

The last equation $PD_5=PS\underset{+}{\circ}(1-SD_P)$ completes the conclusive material that helps us to exclude doubtful diagnoses in the examined patient. After adapting the operation (4.2) to (3.30) we get

$$\mu_{PD_5}(P_1,D_k)=\frac{\sum_{j=1}^{n}\mu_{PS}(P_1,S_j))\cdot(1-\mu_{SD_P}(S_j,D_k))}{\sum_{j=1}^{n}(1-\mu_{SD_P}(S_j,D_k))} \tag{4.9}$$

for $j=1,2,\ldots,n$ and $k=1,2,\ldots,p$.

Let us confirm the validity of newly suggested operations (4.5)–(4.9) by reconsidering the well-known case that concerns the input data of patient $P_1$ from Ex. 3.16.

**Example 4.2**

We use the entries of the same matrices *PS*, $SD_P$ and $SD_D$ that have already been tested in Ex. 3.16, but now we intend to perform the operations on their membership degrees by executing the operations related to (4.5)–(4.9).

The relation $PD_1=PS\underset{+}{\circ}SD_P$, has a component *PS*, accepted according with Ex. 3.8 as

$$\begin{matrix} & & S_1 & S_2 & S_3 & S_4 & S_5 & S_6 & S_7 & S_8 & S_9 & S_{10} & \\ PS = P_1[ & & 1 & 0.515 & 0.913 & 0.653 & 0.345 & 0.632 & 0.720 & 0.9 & 0.0004 & 0.353 & ]. \end{matrix}$$

After the composition of $PS$ with $SD_P$, as recommended by (4.5), we find $PD_1$ in the form of

$$\begin{matrix} & S_1 & S_2 & S_3 & S_4 & S_5 & S_6 & S_7 & S_8 & S_9 & S_{10} & \\ PD_1 = P_1[ & 1 & 0.515 & 0.913 & 0.653 & 0.345 & 0.632 & 0.720 & 0.9 & 0.0004 & 0.353 & ]\underset{+}{\circ} \end{matrix}$$

$$\begin{matrix} & D_1 & D_2 & D_3 \\ S_1 & 0.86 & 0.86 & 0.86 \\ S_2 & 0.016 & 0.25 & 0.938 \\ S_3 & 0.75 & 0.86 & 0.86 \\ S_4 & 0.86 & 0.938 & 0.938 \\ S_5 & 0.016 & 0.86 & 0.938 \\ S_6 & 0.016 & 0.14 & 0.75 \\ S_7 & 0.016 & 0.062 & 0.5 \\ S_8 & 0.938 & 0.86 & 0.86 \\ S_9 & 0.938 & 0.938 & 0.938 \\ S_{10} & 0.86 & 0.75 & 0.75 \end{matrix} = \begin{matrix} & D_1 & D_2 & D_3 \\ P_1[ & 0.624 & 0.591 & 0.593]. \end{matrix}$$

The membership degree of $(P_1, D_1)$ has been induced by computations: $\mu_{PD_1}(P_1, D_1) = (1\cdot0.86+0.515\cdot0.016+0.913\cdot0.75+0.653\cdot0.86+0.345\cdot0.016+0.632\cdot 0.016+0.720\cdot0.016+0.9\cdot0.938+0.0004\cdot0.938+0.353\cdot0.86)/(0.86+0.016+0.75+0.86 +0.016+0.016+0.016+0.938+0.938+0.86) = 3.2899/5.27 = 0.624$.

After employing (4.6) the relation $PD_2$ is decided to be a matrix

$$PD_2 = PS \underset{+}{\circ} SD_D = \begin{matrix} & D_1 & D_2 & D_3 \\ P_1[ & 0.635 & 0.581 & 0.616] \end{matrix} .$$

By utilizing (4.7) we determine the elements of $PD_3$ as a one-row table

$$PD_3 = \text{mean}(PD_1, PD_2) = \begin{matrix} & D_1 & D_2 & D_3 \\ P_1[ & 0.629 & 0.586 & 0.604], \end{matrix}$$

in which the membership degrees distinctly appear as the indicators of a sequence of possible diagnoses taken in the order $D_1$, $D_3$, $D_2$.

In order to confirm the decision made above, let us also consider results of the operations excluding diagnoses. The matrix $PD_4$, calculated by applying of (4.8), is stated as

$$PD_4 = (1 - PS) \underset{+}{\circ} SD_P = \begin{matrix} & D_1 & D_2 & D_3 \\ P_1 & [0.375 & 0.408 & 0.407] \end{matrix}.$$

$PD_4$ clearly provides us with the order of rejected diagnoses. By taking into account the value order among membership degrees in the last relation, we reject diagnoses in $P_1$ in the sequence $D_2$, $D_3$, $D_1$. This still testifies the fact that $D_1$ is the most probable illness typical of these symptoms that have been found and reported by a doctor for $P_1$'s sake.

The entries of $PD_5$ are effects of performed operations in accordance with (4.9). They are written down in the matrix

$$PD_5 = PS \underset{+}{\circ} (1 - SD_P) = \begin{matrix} & D_1 & D_2 & D_3 \\ P_1 & [0.579 & 0.624 & 0.655] \end{matrix}.$$

The numbers still assure that $D_1$ should be assigned to $P_1$ as the most probable diagnosis because of the least value of the membership degree accompanying $D_1$ in the last "rejection" matrix.

The final decision is now submitted in Table 4.1.

Table 4.1: Weighted relation compositions in the diagnostic decision

| Patient | $PD_3$ | | | $PD_4$ | | | $PD_5$ | | | Decision |
|---|---|---|---|---|---|---|---|---|---|---|
| | $D_1$ | $D_2$ | $D_3$ | $D_1$ | $D_2$ | $D_3$ | $D_1$ | $D_2$ | $D_3$ | |
| $P_1$ | 0.629 | 0.586 | 0.604 | 0.375 | 0.408 | 0.407 | 0.579 | 0.624 | 0.655 | $D_1$ |

There is no doubt that $D_1$ satisfies all conditions that the optimal diagnosis should fulfil. The membership degree of $D_1$ in the matrix of acceptance $PD_3$ is the largest of all observed values. The membership degrees of $D_1$ in the matrices of rejection $PD_4$ and $PD_5$ are the smallest that confirm the rules already discussed in Section 3.4.

The next example explains how to use the OWA definition to compute the membership value of one entry belonging to the relation $PD_1$.

**Example 4.3**

The membership degree of ($P_1$, $D_1$), already evaluated in Ex. 4.2, also constitutes a result of the OWA definition expansion (4.1).

If $x_1, x_2, \ldots, x_{10}$ are equal to $\mu_{PS}(P_1, S_1)$, $\mu_{PS}(P_1, S_2)$, …, $\mu_{PS}(P_1, S_{10})$ respectively, then:

- $a_0 = 0$;
- $x_{(1)}$ = min(1, 0.515, 0.913, 0.653, 0.345, 0.632, 0.720, 0.9, 0.0004, 0.353) = 0.0004, which suggests accepting $a_1$ as
$$a_1 = \frac{\mu_{SD_P}(S_9, D_1)}{\mu_{SD_P}(S_1, D_1) + \cdots + \mu_{SD_P}(S_{10}, D_1)} = \frac{0.938}{5.27} \approx 0.178\,;$$
- $x_{(2)}$ = max(min(0.515, 0.913, 0.653, 0.345, 0.632, 0.720, 0.9, 0.0004, 0.353), min(1, 0.913, 0.653, 0.345, 0.632, 0.720, 0.9, 0.0004, 0.353), min(1, 0.515, 0.653, 0.345, 0.632, 0.720, 0.9, 0.0004, 0.353), min(1, 0.515, 0.913, 0.345, 0.632, 0.720, 0.9, 0.0004, 0.353), min(1, 0.515, 0.913, 0.653, 0.632, 0.720, 0.9, 0.0004, 0.353), min(1, 0.515, 0.913, 0.653, 0.345, 0.720, 0.9, 0.0004, 0.353), min(1, 0.515, 0.913, 0.653, 0.345, 0.632, 0.9, 0.0004, 0.353), min(1, 0.515, 0.913, 0.653, 0.345, 0.632, 0.720, 0.0004, 0.353), min(1, 0.515, 0.913, 0.653, 0.345, 0.632, 0.720, 0.9, 0.353), min(1, 0.515, 0.913, 0.653, 0.345, 0.632, 0.720, 0.9, 0.0004)) = max(0.0004, 0.0004, 0.0004, 0.0004, 0.0004, 0.0004, 0.0004, 0.0004, 0.345, 0.0004) = 0.345, which generates
$$a_2 = \frac{\mu_{SD_P}(S_5, D_1)}{\mu_{SD_P}(S_1, D_1) + \cdots + \mu_{SD_P}(S_{10}, D_1)} = \frac{0.016}{5.27} \approx 0.003\,;$$

  ...
- $x_{(10)}$ = max(min(1), min(0.515), min(0.913), min(0.653), min(0.345), min(0.632), min(0.720), min(0.9), min(0.0004), min(0.353)) = 1. The corresponding coefficient $a_{10}$ is a result of the computation
$$a_{10} = \frac{\mu_{SD_P}(S_1, D_1)}{\mu_{SD_P}(S_1, D_1) + \cdots + \mu_{SD_P}(S_{10}, D_1)} = \frac{0.86}{5.27} \approx 0.163\,.$$

Equation (4.1) is used as a basis of the evaluation of the membership degree $\mu_{PD_1}(P_1, D_1) = f(x_1, x_2, ..., x_{10}) = a_0 + a_1 \cdot x_{(1)} + a_2 \cdot x_{(2)} + \cdots + a_{10} \cdot x_{(10)} =$ $0.178 \cdot 0.0004 + 0.003 \cdot 0.345 + \cdots + 0.86 \cdot 1 = 0.624$.

The performed operations in Ex. 4.3 are not recommended to apply in practical cases. We only want to convince a reader that the proposed formula (4.2) is logically correct as a kind of the OWA operation introduced by (4.1).

The use of weighed operations in decision equations (4.5)–(4.9) instead of earlier suggested max-min compositions makes the diagnostic process clearer and more reliable. The differences among membership degrees in decision matrices are large enough to recognize the appropriate diagnosis without making a mistake.

We can conclude that the common influence of all membership degrees, computed in *PS* and *SD*, on values placed in the decision matrices $PD_1$–$PD_5$ improve the quality of a final decision.

Some researchers, who deal with theoretical assumptions of fuzzy set theory, sometimes criticize operations containing computations of mean values. To defend this sort of calculations involved in the diagnostic model we should emphasize that each little change in the symptom index brings valuable information and cannot be lost in the decisive process. The results of operations that resemble mean estimates of some parameters assure that important input data will not disappear.

## 4.3 Fuzzy Set Distances in Diagnostic Decisions

The new operations introduced by the previous section have substantially elucidated the changes made in the diagnostic model to get clear decisions. However, they cannot help when biological parameters measured in a patient indicate a tendency to agree with more diseases than one. We thus observe little differences among membership degree values, or contradictory membership values in matrices $PD_3$, $PD_4$ and $PD_5$ that make the obtained specifications of the patient's data almost unreadable.

We can note that a conception of the metrics is a rather popular tool of investigations in most interdisciplinary fields developed by researchers dealing with fuzzy set theory.

Let us recall the formula for computing a distance between two fuzzy sets [40, 95].

**Definition 4.3**

For two fuzzy sets $A = \{(x_i, \mu_A(x_i))\}$ and $B = \{(x_i, \mu_B(x_i))\}$, determined in the universe $X = \{x_i\}$, $i = 1, \ldots, n$, the Euclidean distance $d(A, B)$ between them is approximated by a formula [40, 95]

$$d(A,B) = \sqrt{\sum_{i=1}^{n}(\mu_A(x_i) - \mu_B(x_i))^2} \, . \tag{4.10}$$

The Euclidean distance $d(A, B)$ maps $[0, 1] \times [0, 1]$ into $R \cup \{0\}$ (the set of non-negative values) and fulfils the following conditions:

1. $d(A, B) \geq 0$,
2. If $A = B$ then $d(A, B) = 0$,
3. $d(A, B) = d(B, A)$,
4. $d(A, C) \leq d(A, B)$" $*$ "$d(B, C)$,

where " $*$ " is a certain operation, e.g., addition.

To comprehend an action of the formula (4.10) we go through a simple example that explains the order of performed operations.

**Example 4.4**

We define two fuzzy sets $A$ and $B$ in the common universe $X = [1, 10]$, where $A = 0.2/3 + 0.5/4 + 0.6/5 + 1/7$ and $B = 0.2/4 + 0.4/6 + 0.6/7 + 1/8 + 0.8/9 + 0.5/10$. At first the distance $d(A, B)$ is pre-evaluated by a number $(d(A,B))^2 = (0.2-0)^2 + (0.5-0.2)^2 + (0.6-0)^2 + (0-0.4)^2 + (1-0.6)^2 + (0-1)^2 + (0-0.8)^2 + (0-0.5)^2 = 2.65$ and afterwards measured by $d(A,B) = \sqrt{2.65} \approx 1.63$.

The concept of a distance between fuzzy sets will be utilized in a diagnostic model in order to improve some decision criteria in doubtful cases. We count on the helpful role of a complementary distance method when analyzing almost equal membership degrees, or opposite values in decision matrices that do not provide us with clear conclusions.

Let us restrict the set of diagnoses $D$ to three diagnoses $D_1$, $D_2$ and $D_3$ to make the following discussion comprehensive in details. The mentioned diagnoses can be found in patient $P$.

Suppose that the fuzzy set [56]

$$AP(PD_3) = 1/(P,D_1) + 1/(P,D_2) + 1/(P,D_3) \tag{4.11}$$

is associated with the state of a total acceptance of each diagnosis. Each value of the membership degree in a one-row "ideal" acceptance relation-matrix, $PD_3$, should be compared to one. This matrix in reality, has other values of membership degrees computed for the symptoms evaluated for any patient $P$. The true set $PD_3$ is generally stated as a fuzzy set (a one-row matrix)

$$PD_3 = \mu_{PD_3}(P,D_1)/(P,D_1) + \mu_{PD_3}(P,D_2)/(P,D_2) + \mu_{PD_3}(P,D_3)/(P,D_3). \tag{4.12}$$

In Fig. 4.1 we draw ellipses to mark membership degrees of the pairs $(P, D_1)$, $(P, D_2)$, $(P, D_3)$ coming from the set $AP(PD_3)$, and we use squares as symbols of genuine membership values found in $PD_3$. Figure 4.1, built artificially for the purpose of making concluding remarks, gives us some hints how to rank diagnoses. Due to an impression given by Fig 4.1 we should place them in order $D_1$, $D_2$, $D_3$.

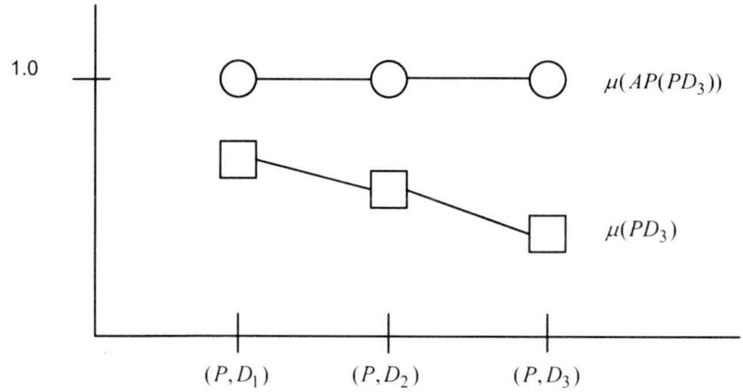


Figure 4.1: The comparison of sets $PD_3$ and $AP(PD_3)$ for patient $P$

Moreover, Fig. 4.1 has another role to fill in; it ought to, via a general image about the distances between real and extreme decision values constructed for $PD_3$, provide us with conclusions that confirm the diagnostic order stated above.

Let us now suppose that we theoretically choose diagnosis $D_1$ with the total security, which introduces the membership degree equal to one in the place of $\mu_{PD_3}(P,D_1)$ in the new set

$$AP(PD_3)_{D_1} = 1/(P,D_1) + \mu_{PD_3}(P,D_2)/(P,D_2) + \mu_{PD_3}(P,D_3)/(P,D_3). \tag{4.13}$$

Analogously, we introduce a set

$$AP(PD_3)_{D_2} = \mu_{PD_3}(P,D_1)/(P,D_1) + 1/(P,D_2) + \mu_{PD_3}(P,D_3)/(P,D_3) \tag{4.14}$$

if we fully adopt $D_2$ in the theoretical way in spite of its real value $\mu_{PD_3}(P,D_2)$.

We also construct a set

$$AP(PD_3)_{D_3} = \mu_{PD_3}(P,D_1)/(P,D_1) + \mu_{PD_3}(P,D_2)/(P,D_2) + 1/(P,D_3) \tag{4.15}$$

that corresponds to the acceptation of diagnosis $D_3$ as a totally true decision.

Let us first visually estimate a distance of $AP(PD_3)_{D_1}$ from $AP(PD_3)$ by regarding the location of theoretically designed membership degrees of both sets in Fig. 4.2. All membership degrees are placed in the same manner as in Fig. 4.1

except for the degree of $D_1$. If $D_1$ is theoretically accepted without any doubts, then the sign marking its membership degree $\mu_{PD_3}(P,D_1)$ in Fig. 4.1 should be removed to such a position in Fig. 4.2, that shows how the membership degree of $AP(PD_3)_{D_1}$ covers the membership degree of $AP(PD_3)$ for the mutual diagnosis $D_1$.

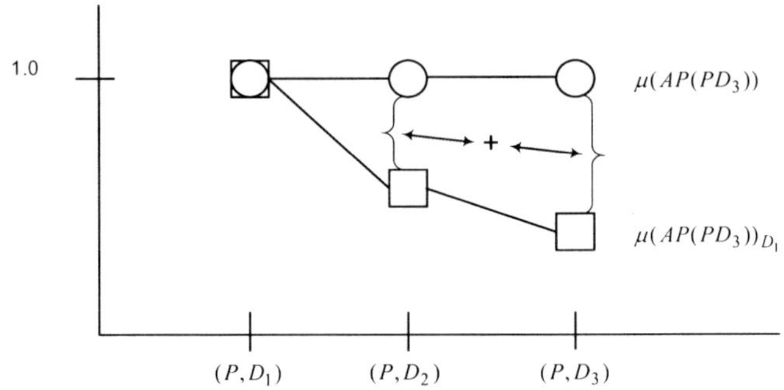


Figure 4.2: The distance between $AP(PD_3)_{D_1}$ and $AP(PD_3)$

To compare some measurements between other characteristic fuzzy sets, we theoretically accept $D_3$ as an absolute diagnosis in $P$. This entails the following changes in Fig. 4.2: we move the membership degree of $D_3$ to the position of one, and return with the membership degree of $D_1$ to the previous location as calculated in $PD_3$. By making the recommended corrections in Fig 4.2, we obtain Fig. 4.3 to evaluate the distance between the sets $AP(PD_3)_{D_3}$ and $AP(PD_3)$.

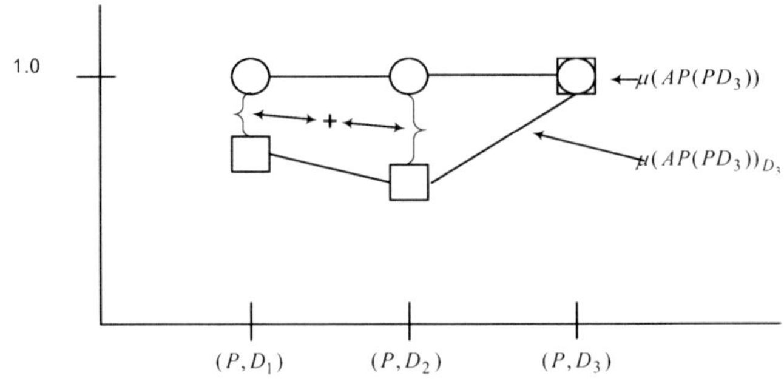


Figure 4.3: The distance between $AP(PD_3)_{D_3}$ and $AP(PD_3)$

The closer analysis of Fig. 4.1, combined with visual estimations of distances revealed by Figs 4.2 and 4.3, provides us with the following conclusion: the larger value of the distance between $AP(PD_3)_{D_k}$, $k = 1, 2, 3$, and $AP(PD_3)$ points to this $D_k$ that possesses the value of one in the set $AP(PD_3)_{D_k}$ as the more truthful diagnosis in $P$.

It is obvious that $D_1$, which has the largest value of all the membership degrees in the set $PD_3$ in accordance with Fig 4.1, is the approved diagnosis in $P$. At the same time the distance of the set $AP(PD_3)_{D_1}$, which is associated with $D_1$, measured from $AP(PD_3)$ is the largest in comparison to other distances with respect to $D_2$ and $D_3$. This finally confirms that $D_1$ should be approved as a recognized illness for $P$.

Let us formulate a conclusion by summing up the premises expressed above.

**Conclusion 4.1**

If the membership degrees in the acceptance matrix $PD_3$ are almost equal or they differ a little from each other, then it will be rather impossible to find a proper diagnosis. We thus recommend an additional method based on distances between fuzzy sets.

We will successively calculate the distances $d_k = d(AP(PD_3), AP(PD_3)_{D_k})$, $k = 1,2,3$, in the case of three diagnoses belonging to the set $D = \{D_1, D_2, D_3\}$. The set $D$ can be extended to as many diagnoses as we can assign to the considered symptoms. We finally approve this $D_k$ that has contributed in the largest value of the distance $d_k$, $k = 1, 2, 3$.

We apply (4.10) to find that

$$d_1 = d(AP(PD_3), AP(PD_3)_{D_1}) = \sqrt{(1-\mu_{PD_3}(P,D_2))^2 + (1-\mu_{PD_3}(P,D_3))^2}\ , \tag{4.16}$$

$$d_2 = d(AP(PD_3), AP(PD_3)_{D_2}) = \sqrt{(1-\mu_{PD_3}(P,D_1))^2 + (1-\mu_{PD_3}(P,D_3))^2} \tag{4.17}$$

and

$$d_3 = d(AP(PD_3), AP(PD_3)_{D_3}) = \sqrt{(1-\mu_{PD_3}(P,D_1))^2 + (1-\mu_{PD_3}(P,D_2))^2}\ . \tag{4.18}$$

To reach a higher grade of accuracy in medical diagnosis, we can also investigate a possibility of rejecting the diagnoses when we still face some unclear data in $PD_3$. If membership degrees in the matrices $PD_4$ and $PD_5$ do not differ essentially from each other, then they will concern us enough to make the best possible decision. To omit this obstacle we propose another diagnostic method based on distances. We preserve $D = \{D_1, D_2, D_3\}$ as a set of diagnoses. Let us introduce two sets

$$JP(PD_4) = \frac{1}{(P,D_1)} + \frac{1}{(P,D_2)} + \frac{1}{(P,D_3)} \tag{4.19}$$

and

$$JP(PD_5) = \frac{1}{(P,D_1)} + \frac{1}{(P,D_2)} + \frac{1}{(P,D_3)}. \tag{4.20}$$

The sets (4.19) and (4.20) correspond to the states of total rejections of all diagnoses in $P$ while the sets $PD_4$ and $PD_5$, constructed for patient $P$, are generally denoted as fuzzy sets (one row-matrices)

$$PD_4 = \frac{\mu_{PD_4}(P,D_1)}{(P,D_1)} + \frac{\mu_{PD_4}(P,D_2)}{(P,D_2)} + \frac{\mu_{PD_4}(P,D_3)}{(P,D_3)} \tag{4.21}$$

and

$$PD_5 = \frac{\mu_{PD_5}(P,D_1)}{(P,D_1)} + \frac{\mu_{PD_5}(P,D_2)}{(P,D_2)} + \frac{\mu_{PD_5}(P,D_3)}{(P,D_3)}. \tag{4.22}$$

Figure 4.4 lets us perceive the range of the distance between true rejection sets and total rejection sets if we preserve the indications (ellipses and squares) introduced in Fig. 4.1.

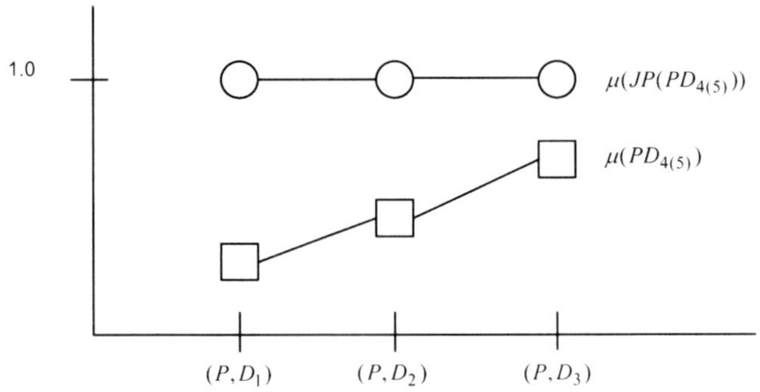


Figure 4.4: The comparison between $PD_4$ (or $PD_5$) and $JP(PD_4)$ (or $JP(PD_5)$)

By following the same way of reasoning as in the case of accepted diagnoses, we consider a secure, theoretical choice of $D_1$. This implies the set $JP(PD_4)_{D_1}$ in which the membership degree of $D_1$ takes the value of one. The set has an appearance as a fuzzy set

$$JP(PD_4)_{D_1} = 1/(P,D_1) + \mu_{PD_4}(P,D_2)/(P,D_2) + \mu_{PD_4}(P,D_3)/(P,D_3). \quad (4.23)$$

Since we are furnished with two matrices of rejection we should also introduce the set $JP(PD_5)_{D_1}$, as a counterpart of $JP(PD_4)_{D_1}$, in the form of

$$JP(PD_5)_{D_1} = 1/(P,D_1) + \mu_{PD_5}(P,D_2)/(P,D_2) + \mu_{PD_5}(P,D_3)/(P,D_3). \quad (4.24)$$

The sets $JP(PD_4)_{D_2}$ and $JP(PD_5)_{D_2}$ correspond to an unquestionable exclusion of $D_2$ and are arranged as

$$JP(PD_4)_{D_2} = \mu_{PD_4}(P,D_1)/(P,D_1) + 1/(P,D_2) + \mu_{PD_4}(P,D_3)/(P,D_3) \quad (4.25)$$

and

$$JP(PD_5)_{D_2} = \mu_{PD_5}(P,D_1)/(P,D_1) + 1/(P,D_2) + \mu_{PD_5}(P,D_3)/(P,D_3). \quad (4.26)$$

Finally, to refuse entirely an existence of $D_3$ we place the value of one as the membership degree of $D_3$ in sets

$$JP(PD_4)_{D_3} = \mu_{PD_4}(P,D_1)/(P,D_1) + \mu_{PD_4}(P,D_2)/(P,D_2) + 1/(P,D_3) \quad (4.27)$$

and

$$JP(PD_5)_{D_3} = \mu_{PD_5}(P,D_1)/(P,D_1) + \mu_{PD_5}(P,D_2)/(P,D_2) + 1/(P,D_3). \quad (4.28)$$

Looking at Fig. 4.4 we experience that the larger value of a distance between $JP(PD_4)_{D_k}$, $k$ = 1, 2, 3, and $JP(PD_4)$ (or $JP(PD_5)_{D_k}$ and $JP(PD_5)$) is related to the more sensible rejection of this $D_k$ that is recognized by the value of one in $JP(PD_4)_{D_k}$ or $JP(PD_5)_{D_k}$.

$D_1$, which now is represented by the smallest value in the rejection matrices $PD_4$ and $PD_5$ according to Fig. 4.4, is still the approved diagnosis for $P$. This holds true because the distance of the set $JP(PD_4)_{D_1}$ from $JP(PD_4)$ (and probably the distance of $JP(PD_5)_{D_1}$ from $JP(PD_5)$) is smallest of all distances computed for $D_2$ and $D_3$ with respect to $JP(PD_{4(5)})_{D_2(D_3)}$ and $JP(PD_{4(5)})$.

We go through the observations that have been made lately and write them down as the following outline.

**Conclusion 4.2**

If the membership degrees in the rejection matrices $PD_4$ and $PD_5$ differ a little from each other, or they induce a contraposition in the diagnostic exclusion, then we will experience difficulties in pointing out some rejected diagnoses. In spite of this inconvenience we supply the next trial of the model improvement still based on distances between fuzzy sets.

We estimate a sequence of distances $d_k^{'} = d(JP(PD_4), JP(PD_4)_{D_k})$, $k = 1,2,3$, (or $d_k^{''} = d(JP(PD_5), JP(PD_5)_{D_k})$) for three diagnoses belonging to set $D = \{D_1, D_2, D_3\}$ (the number of $D$'s members can be definitely enlarged). We reject this $D_k$, which has the largest value of the distance $d_k^{'}$ (or $d_k^{''}$), $k = 1, 2, 3$.

Let us derive formulas for making calculations of distances. We introduce quantities of

$$d_1^{'} = d(JP(PD_4), JP(PD_4)_{D_1}) = \sqrt{(1-\mu_{PD_4}(P,D_2))^2 + (1-\mu_{PD_4}(P,D_3))^2}\,, \tag{4.29}$$

$$d_2^{'} = d(JP(PD_4), JP(PD_4)_{D_2}) = \sqrt{(1-\mu_{PD_4}(P,D_1))^2 + (1-\mu_{PD_4}(P,D_3))^2}\,, \tag{4.30}$$

$$d_3^{'} = d(JP(PD_4), JP(PD_4)_{D_3}) = \sqrt{(1-\mu_{PD_4}(P,D_1))^2 + (1-\mu_{PD_4}(P,D_2))^2} \tag{4.31}$$

as well as

$$d_1^{''} = d(JP(PD_5), JP(PD_5)_{D_1}) = \sqrt{(1-\mu_{PD_5}(P,D_2))^2 + (1-\mu_{PD_5}(P,D_3))^2}\,, \tag{4.32}$$

$$d_2'' = d(JP(PD_5), JP(PD_5)_{D_2}) = \sqrt{(1-\mu_{PD_5}(P,D_1))^2 + (1-\mu_{PD_5}(P,D_3))^2} \quad (4.33)$$

and

$$d_3'' = d(JP(PD_5), JP(PD_5)_{D_3}) = \sqrt{(1-\mu_{PD_5}(P,D_1))^2 + (1-\mu_{PD_5}(P,D_2))^2} \; . \quad (4.34)$$

To make a final decision regarding a choice of the most probable diagnosis in vague decision circumstances we should elaborate the analysis of all obtained distances in accordance with the following criteria:

1. We agree to this diagnosis $D_k$, for which the distance $d_k$, $k = 1, 2, 3$ (generally $k = 1, 2, \ldots, p$) is largest;
2. We neglect this diagnosis $D_k$, that influences the distance $d_k'$ or $d_k''$ to be the largest value for $k = 1, 2, 3$ (generally $k = 1, 2, \ldots, p$).

The method based on distances assists the diagnostic model projected for the next patient $P_3$, whose indices fit for all adequate diagnoses that have been associated with a collection of chosen symptoms.

**Example 4.5**

We assume that patient $P_3$ suffers from one of the diagnoses that have already been investigated in Ex. 3.16. The examinations of ten symptoms, listed in Ex. 3.1, have been converted to the values of membership degrees that constitute the contents of the one-row matrix *PS*. We exploit the formulas (4.5)–(4.9) to make the necessary computations collected in Table 4.2.

Table 4.2: The diagnostic decision concerning patient $P_3$

| Patient | $PD_3$ | | | $PD_4$ | | | $PD_5$ | | | Decision |
|---|---|---|---|---|---|---|---|---|---|---|
| | $D_1$ | $D_2$ | $D_3$ | $D_1$ | $D_2$ | $D_3$ | $D_1$ | $D_2$ | $D_3$ | |
| $P_3$ | 0.755 | 0.795 | 0.62 | 0.3 | 0.62 | 0.755 | 0.82 | 0.41 | 0.41 | *unknown* |

By taking into consideration the membership degrees in $PD_3$, we are able to assign to $P_3$ either a $D_1$ or $D_2$ since they have the largest membership degrees. With respect to $PD_4$ we should exclude $D_3$ and $D_2$ because they show the largest in magnitude degrees. However, this contradicts the results obtained in $PD_5$ where $D_1$ ought to be rejected since its membership degree is largest of all. We have come to contradictory conclusions that make $P_3$'s diagnostic problem unsolvable.

In order to improve the data's decisive character we estimate the distances $d_k$, $d_k^{'}$ and $d_k^{''}$, $k = 1, 2, 3$. Table 4.3 now consists of the revised specification of $P$'s health conditions.

Table 4.3: The distances $d_k$, $d_k^{'}$ and $d_k^{''}$, $k = 1, 2, 3$, evaluated for patient $P_3$

| Patient | $D_1$ | | | $D_2$ | | | $D_3$ | | | Decision |
|---|---|---|---|---|---|---|---|---|---|---|
| | $d_1$ | $d_1^{'}$ | $d_1^{''}$ | $d_2$ | $d_2^{'}$ | $d_2^{''}$ | $d_3$ | $d_3^{'}$ | $d_3^{''}$ | |
| $P_3$ | 0.43 | 0.45 | 0.83 | 0.45 | 0.74 | 0.61 | 0.32 | 0.8 | 0.61 | $D_1$ |

Having compared $d_1$, $d_2$ and $d_3$ we can admit to a placement of $D_1$ or $D_2$ at the top of a hierarchy ladder of the considered diagnoses. The revision of $d_1^{'}$, $d_2^{'}$ and $d_3^{'}$ gives us a tool for deciding that $D_2$ and $D_3$, as the diagnoses with the largest rejection distances $d_2^{'}$ and $d_3^{'}$, are not taken into consideration anymore as possible diagnoses in $P_3$. The numbers $d_1^{''}$, $d_2^{''}$ and $d_3^{''}$ do not vary from each other in the substantial grade anymore, which allows us to omit their influence on the final decision. Since $D_1$ is characterized by the essential low value of $d_1^{'}$, and by the substantial high value of $d_1$ then we can take a risk of choosing this diagnosis as a primary diagnosis in the patient. The choice is confirmed by the experienced physician who has examined $P_3$.

The distance method of diagnosing can be helpful in cases that contain hardly interpretable or vague decision data, but we can imagine that a physician should obtain better diagnostic results after more than one examination of a patient. Some wider and richer reports of symptom observations can prevent a diagnostician from making a mistake when the clinical state of a patient shows a tendency to some changes.

## 4.4 Diagnostic Processes Extended in Time Intervals

This section refers to earlier results obtained in Chapter 3 and Section 4.2 and constitutes their essential complement and extension. A new assumption aims at the introduction of repeated medical examinations in which measurements of symptoms are regularly made. In this way we can render all essential changes in symptom values resulting in making an appropriate diagnostic decision. The model offered below concerns the observations of symptoms in an individual patient at a time interval.

The behaviour of the symptoms over a period of time, conduces to the access of some additional information. This sometimes is very important in a diagnostic process in which several clinical pictures of a patient, obtained during a certain time interval, differ from each other and point to different diagnoses. It may occur that the change in the intensity of a symptom decides an acceptance of another diagnosis, when, after some time, the patient does not feel better.

The objective now is to fix an optimal diagnosis on the basis of clinical symptoms typical of several diagnoses with respect to the changes of these symptoms throughout time. Both the intensity of some symptoms, and the retreat of another group of them observed during a certain specific period of time, constitutes an additional factor that supports the selection of a diagnosis.

In order to solve a diagnostic model extended in time, we again modify fuzzy relation equations as discussed in Subsections 3.4 and 4.2. Moreover, in the final decision concerning the choice of an adequate diagnosis, the adoption of a normalized Euclidean distance is suggested as a measure between an objective decision and an "ideal" decision. As usual we check the relevance of the model by testing some sampled clinical data.

We consider three non-fuzzy sets representing only one patient [56, 58, 61]:

1. A set of *"stages of observations"* $T = \{T_1, T_2, \ldots, T_m\}$, where each symbol $T_i$, $i = 1, 2, \ldots, m$, stands for a new phase of the examination;
2. A set of symptoms $S = \{S_1, S_2, \ldots, S_n\}$ in which each biological symptom-parameter $S_j$, $j = 1, 2, \ldots, n$, has been described or measured in the successive examination $T_i$;
3. A set of diagnoses $D = \{D_1, D_2, \ldots, D_p\}$, where to each diagnosis $D_k$, $k = 1, 2, \ldots, p$, one may assign the symptoms occurring in the set $S$.

Each of the symptoms $S_j \in S$, $j = 1, 2, \ldots, n$, is a fuzzy set with the membership function being modelled according to a kind of symptom (see Section 3.3) and allowing one to assign the membership degree to a fix value of this symptom.

The *"stage – symptom"* fuzzy relation formed as a collection of membership degrees of the pairs $(T_i, S_j)$, $i = 1, 2, \ldots, m$, $j = 1, 2, \ldots, n$, is written down as a matrix

$$TPS = \begin{array}{c} \\ T_1 \\ T_2 \\ \vdots \\ T_m \end{array} \begin{array}{c} \begin{array}{cccc} \quad S_1 \quad & \quad S_2 \quad & \cdots & \quad S_n \quad \end{array} \\ \begin{bmatrix} \mu_{TPS}(T_1,S_1) & \mu_{TPS}(T_1,S_2) & \cdots & \mu_{TPS}(T_1,S_n) \\ \mu_{TPS}(T_2,S_1) & \mu_{TPS}(T_2,S_2) & \cdots & \mu_{TPS}(T_2,S_n) \\ \vdots & \vdots & \ddots & \vdots \\ \mu_{TPS}(T_m,S_1) & \mu_{TPS}(T_m,S_2) & \cdots & \mu_{TPS}(T_m,S_n) \end{bmatrix} \end{array} . \tag{4.35}$$

The fuzzy relation $1 - TPS$ introduced by a membership function

$$\mu_{1-TPS}(T_i, S_j) = 1 - \mu_{TPS}(T_i, S_j) \tag{4.36}$$

is one of components taking part in decision equations.

We now focus on the presence of symptom $S_j$ in diagnosis $D_k$ on one hand, and on the other hand, the decisive character of $S_j$ for $D_k$ so as to allow one to judge the intensity of a relationship between the symptoms $S_j$ and the diagnoses $D_k$. To each pair ($S_j$, $D_k$) we assign two membership degrees fixed for the linguistic variables "*presence*" and "*decisive character*" (see Subsection 3.4.1). By employing the technique already described in Subsection 3.4.2, we insert two fuzzy relations of "*medical knowledge*" listed as

$$SD_P = \begin{array}{c} \\ S_1 \\ \vdots \\ S_n \end{array} \begin{array}{c} D_1 \quad \cdots \quad D_p \\ \left[ \begin{array}{c} \\ \mu_{\text{"presence"}}(S_j, D_k) \\ \\ \end{array} \right] \end{array} \tag{4.37}$$

and

$$SD_D = \begin{array}{c} \\ S_1 \\ \vdots \\ S_n \end{array} \begin{array}{c} D_1 \quad \cdots \quad D_p \\ \left[ \begin{array}{c} \\ \mu_{\substack{\text{"decisive} \\ \text{character"}}}(S_j, D_k) \\ \\ \end{array} \right] \end{array}. \tag{4.38}$$

The fuzzy relations (4.35), (4.37) and (4.38) are elements of equations yielding relations *TPD* standing for connections "*stage – diagnosis*". These consist of pairs ($T_i$, $D_k$), $i = 1, 2, \ldots, m$, $k = 1, 2, \ldots, p$. By superposing the fuzzy relations *TPS* with $SD_P$ or $SD_D$ with respect to the operation "$\underset{+}{\circ}$" we reproduce the membership functions of relations *TPD* in accordance with the general formula

$$\mu_{TPD}(T_i, D_k) = \frac{\sum_{j=1}^{n} \mu_{TPS}(T_i, S_j) \cdot \mu_{SD}(S_j, D_k)}{\sum_{j=1}^{n} \mu_{SD}(S_j, D_k)} \tag{4.39}$$

for $i = 1, \ldots, m$, $j = 1, \ldots, n$ and $k = 1, \ldots, p$.

The inference rule *modus ponens* (cited in Subsections 3.2 and 3.4) induces an interpretation:

"If the symptom $S_j$ emerges in stage $T_i$ with the membership degree $\mu_{TPS}(T_i, S_j)$"

and

"If the appearance of $S_j$ results in $D_k$ with the membership degree $\mu_{SD_P}(S_j, D_k)$ or $\mu_{SD_D}(S_j, D_k)$"

then
"The diagnosis $D_k$ occurs in the stage $T_i$ with the general membership degree $\mu_{TPD}(T_i, D_k)$".

On the basis of the rule above we will consider a fuzzy relation equation

$$TPD_1 = TPS \underset{+}{\circ} SD_P \tag{4.40}$$

as well as

$$TPD_2 = TPS \underset{+}{\circ} SD_D \,. \tag{4.41}$$

The relations $TPD_1$ and $TPD_2$ are parts of a mean rule leading to

$$TPD_3 = mean(TPD_1, TPD_2)\,, \tag{4.42}$$

provided that the relation $TPD_3$ is a crucial factor deciding the final acceptance of an optimal diagnosis after each examination $T_1, \ldots, T_m$.

An acceptance criterion for the diagnosis $S_j$ at the stage $T_i$ is the same as the conclusion stated in Section 3.4, i.e., the higher membership degree of the diagnosis $D_k$ at the stage $T_i$ corresponds to the more certain approval of $D_k$.

It can happen that the membership degrees in the row $T_i$ of the relation $TPD_3$ (i.e., at the stage $T_i$) differ a little and do not indicate the optimal diagnosis as a clear-cut decision. Therefore it is also recommended to inspect an opportunity of rejecting the diagnosis.

Another rule of inference *modus tollens*, already familiar to us, creates a foundation for the statement:
"If the symptom $S_j$ does not appear in stage $T_i$ with the membership degree $1 - \mu_{TPS}(T_i, S_j)$"
and
"It is true that $D_k$ requires presence of $S_j$ with the membership degree $\mu_{SD_P}(S_j, D_k)$"
then
"The diagnosis $D_k$ is rejected in the patient at the stage $T_i$ with the membership degree $\mu_{TPD}(T_i, D_k)$".

The above interpretation of the *modus tollens* law involved in the diagnosis exclusion gives rise to setting the next fuzzy relation equation

$$TPD_4 = (1 - TPS) \underset{+}{\circ} SD_P \,. \tag{4.43}$$

By proving a modification of the same logical *modus tollens* law, we formulate the next equation as the compound operation involving the relations $TPS$ and $1 - SD_P$ in a relation

$$TPD_5 = TPS \underset{+}{\circ} (1 - SD_P) . \tag{4.44}$$

The fuzzy relations $TPD_4$ and $TPD_5$ play an essential role in the rejecting of inadequate diagnoses at the successive stages $T_i$, $i = 1, \ldots, m$. The higher the membership degree value of $D_k$ at the $T_i$ stage in $TPD_4$ and $TPD_5$, the greater the certainty that the $D_k$-diagnosis will be rejection. All the conclusions are valid for $i = 1, 2, \ldots, m, j = 1, 2, \ldots, n$ and $k = 1, 2, \ldots, p$.

The final decision concerning the acceptance of the proper diagnosis assumes a thorough analysis of the entire period of observations at the stages $T_1, T_2, \ldots, T_m$. The hierarchy of diagnoses during this period of time in a considered patient is established by the estimation of the Euclidean distances between fuzzy sets.

Each diagnosis $D_k$, $k = 1, 2, \ldots, p$ occurring as the $k^{\text{th}}$ column in the relations $TPD_t$ ("*stage – diagnosis*"), $t = 1, 2, 3, 4, 5$, is interpreted as a fuzzy set

$$D_k = {\mu_{TPD_t}(T_1, D_k)}/{T_1} + {\mu_{TPD_t}(T_2, D_k)}/{T_2} + \cdots + {\mu_{TPD_t}(T_m, D_k)}/{T_m} . \tag{4.45}$$

Let us demonstrate an uncomplicated example to make an interpretation of the set $D_k$ a bit easier.

**Example 4.6**

We consider three diagnoses $D_1, D_2, D_3$ in a relation $TPD_1$, computed for four stages of symptom observations. The relation $TPD_1$, written down as the matrix

$$TPD_1 = \begin{array}{c} \\ T_1 \\ T_2 \\ T_3 \\ T_4 \end{array} \begin{array}{c} \begin{array}{ccc} D_1 & D_2 & D_3 \end{array} \\ \begin{bmatrix} 0.7 & 0.3 & 0.6 \\ 0.6 & 0.5 & 0.5 \\ 0.8 & 0.4 & 0.3 \\ 0.5 & 0.2 & 0.3 \end{bmatrix} \end{array} ,$$

introduces diagnosis $D_1$ as the fuzzy set

$$D_1 = {\mu_{TPD_1}(T_1, D_1)}/{T_1} + {\mu_{TPD_1}(T_2, D_1)}/{T_2} + {\mu_{TPD_1}(T_3, D_1)}/{T_3} + {\mu_{TPD_1}(T_4, D_1)}/{T_4}$$

or, more specifically, as the set $D_1 = 0.7/T_1 + 0.6/T_2 + 0.8/T_3 + 0.5/T_4$ .

A set of "total acceptance" or "total rejection" of diagnosis $D_k$ on the basis of observed symptoms at stages $T_1, \ldots, T_m$, is assumed to be the set given by

$$D = {}^{1}\!/_{T_1} + {}^{1}\!/_{T_2} + \cdots + {}^{1}\!/_{T_m} \tag{4.46}$$

because the membership degree of the fully accepted diagnosis $D_k$ in the relation $TPD_3$ and the totally rejected diagnosis in $TPD_4$ and $TPD_5$, when considering each stage, should be equal to the rarely achieved value "*one*".

The distance of the set $D_k$ from the set $D$ is estimated by applying the Euclidean normalized distance

$$e_k = e(D_k, D) = \sqrt{\frac{1}{m}\sum_{i=1}^{m}(\mu_{TPD_t}(T_i, D_k) - 1)^2}\ , \tag{4.47}$$

for $t = 3, 4, 5$ and $k = 1, \ldots, p$.

It is easy to conclude that there exist some relationships between magnitudes of the distances $e_k$ estimated for $D_k$ and the decisions of its acceptance or rejection from a set of diagnoses possible in a patient. The smaller the distance from the set $D$ to the fuzzy set $D_k$, created in $TPD_3$, the stronger the acceptance of the diagnosis $D_k$ will be assumed in the considered patient. A similar conclusion concerns the diagnoses forming the columns of the relations $TPD_4$ and $TPD_5$, i.e., the small distance of $D_k$ from set $D$ that indicates the excluded illness in a patient.

It ought to appear a theoretical connection, e.g., for two diagnoses $D_1$ and $D_2$:

a) If $D_1$ is the accepted diagnosis, then $D_1$ tends to have the smaller distance $e(D_1, D)$ than $e(D_2, D)$, for $D_1$, $D_2$ taken as the columns in $TPD_3$.

b) If $D_2$ is the rejected diagnosis, then $D_2$ shows the smaller distance $e(D_2, D)$ than $e(D_1, D)$, for $D_1$, $D_2$ appearing as the columns in $TPD_4$ and $TPD_5$.

The next medical sample of data is tested to prove the successful action of observations throughout time.

**Example 4.7**

The relation *TPS*, built for patient $P_1$, collects the membership degrees assigned to his symptom values that have been estimated three times during separate visits at the hospital. We introduce *TPS* as the matrix

$$PS = \begin{matrix} \\ T_1 \\ T_2 \\ T_3 \end{matrix} \begin{matrix} S_1 & S_2 & S_3 & S_4 & S_5 & S_6 & S_7 & S_8 & S_9 & S_{10} \\ \end{matrix} \begin{bmatrix} 1 & 0.515 & 0.913 & 0.653 & 0.345 & 0.632 & 0.720 & 0.9 & 0.0004 & 0.353 \\ 1 & 0.875 & 0.523 & 0.569 & 0.543 & 0.576 & 0.641 & 0.7 & 0.0008 & 0.342 \\ 1 & 0.712 & 0.320 & 0.436 & 0.634 & 0.543 & 0.436 & 0.6 & 0.0005 & 0.326 \end{bmatrix}.$$

We note that the patient has improved the values of some unfavourable parameters like smoking, hypertension and lack of physical activity after his first consultation with a doctor. We can imagine that $P_1$ has taken the doctor's advice into serious consideration.

By using Eqs (4.40)–(4.42) we compute membership degrees of the relation $TPD_3$ whereas Eqs (4.43) and (4.44) give rise to $TPD_4$ and $TPD_5$. All relations are demonstrated in Table 4.4.

Table 4.4: The relations $TPD_3$, $TPD_4$ and $TPD_5$ made for $P_1$

| Stage | $TPD_3$ | | | $TPD_4$ | | | $TPD_5$ | | | Decision |
|---|---|---|---|---|---|---|---|---|---|---|
| | $D_1$ | $D_2$ | $D_3$ | $D_1$ | $D_2$ | $D_3$ | $D_1$ | $D_2$ | $D_3$ | |
| $T_1$ | 0.629 | 0.586 | 0.604 | 0.376 | 0.408 | 0.407 | 0.579 | 0.625 | 0.655 | $D_1$ |
| $T_2$ | 0.520 | 0.539 | 0.583 | 0.481 | 0.462 | 0.426 | 0.641 | 0.649 | 0.590 | $D_3$ |
| $T_3$ | 0.445 | 0.485 | 0.510 | 0.553 | 0.519 | 0.497 | 0.560 | 0.539 | 0.488 | $D_3$ |

The final decision, pointing out a right diagnosis, is rather clear on the basis of clinical symptoms observed during each distinct visit at the doctor's. Let us prove the distance method according to (4.47) that helps us to weigh intensities of the examined symptoms in time. To carry out the comparison of all involved distances we place the obtained results in Table 4.5.

Table 4.5: The final acceptance of diagnosis by means of distances

| Patient | $TPD_3$ | | | $TPD_4$ | | | $TPD_5$ | | | Decision |
|---|---|---|---|---|---|---|---|---|---|---|
| | $e_1$ | $e_2$ | $e_3$ | $e_1$ | $e_2$ | $e_3$ | $e_1$ | $e_2$ | $e_3$ | |
| $P_1$ | 0.474 | 0.465 | 0.436 | 0.534 | 0.539 | 0.558 | 0.408 | 0.398 | 0.428 | $D_3$ |

To explain the procedure of computing the membership degrees that are the results of (4.47), we go through a basic example of executing the necessary operations to get $e_1$ in $TPD_3$ as $e_1 = \sqrt{\frac{1}{3}\left((0.629-1)^2 + (0.520-1)^2 + (0.445-1)^2\right)} = 0.474$.

We should reject $D_1$ and $D_2$ on the basis of the relations $TPD_4$ and $TPD_5$ for which $e_1$ and $e_2$ are the smallest values. The value $e_3$ computed for $TPD_3$ as the smallest of all confirms that $D_3$ should be recognized for $P_1$'s sake. We thus decide that $P_1$, who has suffered from $D_1$ at the first examination stage, actually runs the high risk of going down with $D_3$ (infarct) if he is not careful enough and does not improve risk factors in his parameters.

The proposed method for establishing the correct diagnosis on the basis of clinical symptoms *observed in time*, constitutes an essential improvement of the diagnostic process because it optimizes the diagnosing by correction and verification of decisions with respect being paid to the variability of symptoms in time. The changes in intensities of symptom presence at some time influence not only a choice of the most appropriate diagnosis, but also affect a rejection of less accurate diseases.

## 4.5 Rough Set Theory in the Classification of Diagnoses

Rough set theory is a new mathematical approach to intelligent data analysis and data mining [50, 51, 52, 53].

Rough set philosophy is founded on the assumption that some information is associated with every object of the considered universe set. The objects characterized by the same information are indiscernible (similar) in view of the available information about them. The indiscernibility relation generated for similar objects is the mathematical basis of rough set theory. Any set of similar objects, being the equivalence class of the similarity relation, is called an elementary set. Any union of some elementary sets (equivalence classes) is a crisp set (a precise set). Such union of elementary sets, which has boundary-line cases, i.e., objects that cannot be classified with certainty, constitutes a rough set (an imprecise, vague set).

With any rough set, a pair of precise sets – called a lower and an upper approximation of the rough set – is associated. The lower approximation consists of all objects that surely belong to the set, and the upper approximation contains all objects that possibly belong to the set. A difference between the upper and the lower approximation constitutes the boundary region of the rough set. Approximations are two basic operations in the rough set theory.

Let us first introduce the theoretical background of rough sets and afterwards let us prove their usefulness via presenting a practical problem concerning medical diagnosing. All conceptions and annotations will be accommodated to a medical model to make it easier at the stage of practical interpretation.

We start with an information system constructed as a data table whose columns are labelled by attributes. Objects of interest label the table rows, and entries of the table are attribute values. In a new scenario of the diagnostic discussion, interpreted now as a classification of diagnoses, we adopt the set of patients $P = \{P_1, \ldots, P_m\}$ with objects $P_i$, $i = 1, \ldots, m$, as a *universe set* $P$. The set of *condition attributes* $S$ is established as a set of symptoms $S = \{S_1, \ldots, S_n\}$. With every attribute $S_j \in S$, $j = 1, \ldots, n$, we associate a set $V_{S_j} = \{x_{S_j}^1, x_{S_j}^2, \ldots, x_{S_j}^{t(S_j)}\}$ of its values, called the *domain* of $S_j$. In the diagnostic problem the set $V_{S_j}$ will contain some linguistic terms or values of the membership degrees of $S_j$ expressed by codes that correspond to the intensity grades of $S_j$. Any subset $B$ of $S$ determines a binary relation $I(B)$ on $B$, which will be called an *indiscernibility* relation. The relation $I(B)$ is defined by an inclusion operation

$$(P_i, P_l) \in I(B) \text{ if } S_j(P_i) = S_j(P_l), \tag{4.48}$$

for each $S_j \in B \subseteq S$, $i$, $l = 1, \ldots, m$, $j = 1, \ldots, n$, where $S_j(P_i)$ denotes the value $x_{S_j}^c$, $c = 1, \ldots, t(S_j)$, of attribute $S_j$ for the element $P_i$.

The relation $I(B)$ is *reflexive* because $(P_i, P_i) \in I(B) \leftrightarrow S_j(P_i) = S_j(P_i)$ for each $P_i \in P$.

Since $(P_i, P_l) \in I(B) \leftrightarrow S_j(P_i) = S_j(P_l) \leftrightarrow S_j(P_l) = S_j(P_i) \leftrightarrow (P_l, P_i) \in I(B)$ for $P_i$, $P_l \in I(B)$, then $I(B)$ will be a *symmetric* relation, too.

Finally, the assumptions $(P_i, P_l) \in I(B)$ and $(P_l, P_r) \in I(B)$ for $P_i$, $P_l$, $P_r \in P$ imply $S_j(P_i) = S_j(P_r) \leftrightarrow (P_i, P_r) \in I(B)$. $I(B)$ thus is a *transitive* relation.

The sign "↔" is interpreted as "which is equivalent to".

For the reason of such properties as reflexivity, symmetry and transitivity $I(B)$ is recognized as an equivalence relation.

It is possible to make a partition of the set $P$, with respect to $B$, by means of the relation $I(B)$ to obtain equivalence classes $IB(P_i)$ defined by

$$IB(P_i) = \{P_l : (P_i, P_l) \in I(B)\}, \tag{4.49}$$

for each $i$, $l = 1, \ldots, m$. The classes $IB(P_i)$ are additionally called elementary sets. We realize that these sets contain the objects $P_i$, which are identical, i.e., in the considered case, they gather patients who suffer from a presence of the same symptoms characterized by the same intensity.

The symptoms $S_j$ constitute the condition attributes in the diagnostic model. Besides these, we also consider a decision attribute – the diagnosis $D_1$. $D_1$ has a set of values determined as "*yes*" if it is found in the patient, "*no*" if the patient is free from it and "*unknown*" when a decision about the presence of the diagnosis cannot be clearly formulated.

By resuming the assumptions made so far we can come to a conclusion that the contents of the classification table, giving rise to the indiscernibility relation $I(B)$, corresponds to a *triple* $(P, S, D_1)$ in the model of diagnoses. The patients $P_i$ are placed in the first column of the table, the three values of $D_1$ appear in the last column while the rest of the table positions are filled with the values of condition attributes.

The aim of the classification, accomplished by $I(B)$ or rather its equivalence classes, is to divide the patients belonging to $P$ in three groups. These three groups are; a group of patients who surely are ill with $D_1$, a sample of patients who may suffer from $D_1$ and a collection of patients who do not have diagnosis $D_1$.

Let us create a set $P_{yes} \subseteq P$ in accordance with the following definition

$$P_{yes} = \{P_i : D_1 \text{ has decision "}yes\text{" assigned}\}, \tag{4.50}$$

for $i = 1, \ldots, m$.

We now state two sets surrounded $P_{yes} \subseteq P$ that are treated as its lower and upper approximations.

The lower approximation $B_*(P_{yes})$ of $P_{yes}$ is built by an inclusion operator as

$$B_*(P_{yes}) = \{P_i : IB(P_i) \subseteq P_{yes}\} \tag{4.51}$$

and rendered as a set of these $P_i$ that have $D_1$ assigned with a full security.

Another set, the upper approximation $B^*(P_{yes})$ of $P_{yes}$ is designed by

$$B^*(P_{yes}) = \{P_i : IB(P_i) \cap P_{yes} \neq 0\} \tag{4.52}$$

and accepted as a sampling of those objects $P_i$ that possibly are members of the class $D_1$ possessing the attribute "*yes*" ($D_1$ = "*yes*").

The set $P_{yes}$ is thus bounded by two sets in compliance with the inclusion $B_*(P_{yes}) \subseteq P_{yes} \subseteq B^*(P_{yes})$ and referred to the approximation sets as rough or inexact with respect to $B$.

Even a boundary set

$$B_{border}(P_{yes}) = B^*(P_{yes}) - B_*(P_{yes}) \tag{4.53}$$

contains some useful information about the objects that are uncertain members of the class $D_1$ = "*yes*".

To measure a grade of membership uncertainty in $D_1$ = "*yes*" for each $P_i$, we recommend applying the formula for computing membership degrees

$$\mu_{D_1="yes"}(P_i) = \frac{|P_{yes} \cap IB(P_i)|}{|IB(P_i)|}, \tag{4.54}$$

in which the symbol "$|\ |$" denotes the cardinality of a set (the number of elements belonging to a set).

A selection of the $B$-subset of $S$ should be made with the special care to assure good classification results. We can measure a coefficient $\alpha_B$ called the accuracy of approximation in conformity with

$$\alpha_B(P_{yes}) = \frac{|B_*(P_{yes})|}{|B^*(P_{yes})|} \tag{4.55}$$

to measure an adaptation grade of $B$ to the decision table ($P$, $S$, $D_1$).

We demonstrate the utility of rough sets in the diagnosis classification process by studying steps of the following example.

**Example 4.8**

In Ex. 3.1 we have already listed 10 symptoms that are the elements of the set of symptoms $S$. Let us select set $B \subseteq S$ as $B = \{S_3, S_4, S_8, S_9, S_{10}\}$. Set $B$ contains the most significant symptoms that are characteristic of diagnosis $D_1$.

We now prepare sets of values corresponding to the selected symptoms.

Since $S_3$ and $S_4$ are compound qualitative parameters measured by means of a questionnaire, then we can place their membership degrees in the continuous interval [0, 1]. The quantitative indicators $S_8$, $S_9$ and $S_{10}$ possess the same property. In order to vary some intensity grades of the symptoms' appearance as discrete characteristic quantities, we construct the following codes associated with the membership values $\mu_{S_j}(P_i)$, $j = 3, 4, 8, 9, 10$, belonging to subintervals of [0, 1]. We assign the code 0 to $\mu_{S_j}(P_i) \in [0, 0.25)$, 1 – to $\mu_{S_j}(P_i) \in [0.25, 0.5)$, 2 – to $\mu_{S_j}(P_i) \in [0.5, 0.75)$ and, finally, 3 – to $\mu_{S_j}(P_i) \in [0.75, 1]$. The codes generate sets $V_{S_j} = \{0,1,2,3\}$, $j = 3, 4, 8, 9, 10$.

Suppose that $P = \{P_1, P_2, P_3, P_4, P_5, P_6\}$. The patients $P_1$, $P_2$, $P_5$ suffer from $D_1$, $P_3$, $P_6$ have $D_2$ assigned and the diagnosis concerning $D_4$ is unknown. We decide the members of set $P_{yes} = \{P_1, P_2, P_5\}$. To regard $P_{yes}$ as rough, we should find its lower and upper approximation. In this way we count on classifying the unknown object $P_4$.

By assuming that the knowledge of clinical symptoms is absolutely correct, we fill in Table 4.6 known as $(P, S, D_1)$ that constitutes a basis for establishing an indiscernibility relation $I(B)$.

Table 4.6: The table $(P, S, D_1)$ in diagnosis classification

| Patients | Codes characteristic of symptoms | | | | | Decision about $D_1$ |
|---|---|---|---|---|---|---|
| | $S_3$ | $S_4$ | $S_8$ | $S_9$ | $S_{10}$ | |
| $P_1$ | 1 | 1 | 2 | 1 | 2 | *yes* |
| $P_2$ | 2 | 3 | 1 | 2 | 3 | *yes* |
| $P_3$ | 2 | 2 | 2 | 3 | 1 | *no* |
| $P_4$ | 2 | 3 | 1 | 2 | 3 | *unknown* |
| $P_5$ | 1 | 2 | 2 | 2 | 2 | *yes* |
| $P_6$ | 1 | 1 | 3 | 2 | 1 | *no* |

The relation $I(B)$ consists of the pairs of patients $(P_i, P_l)$, $i, l = 1, \ldots, 6$, which when comparing rows $i$ and $l$, all have equal codes.

We list $I(B)$ as $I(B) = \{(P_1, \mathrm{P}_1), (P_2, \mathrm{P}_2), (P_3, \mathrm{P}_3), (P_4, \mathrm{P}_4), (P_5, \mathrm{P}_5), (P_6, \mathrm{P}_6), (P_2, \mathrm{P}_4), (P_4, \mathrm{P}_2)\}$. The elementary sets of $I(B)$ or its equivalent classes are given as the sets $IB(P_1) = \{P_1\}$, $IB(P_2) = \{P_2, \mathrm{P}_4\}$, $IB(P_3) = \{P_3\}$, $IB(P_4) = \{P_2, \mathrm{P}_4\}$, $IB(P_5) = \{P_5\}$, $IB(P_6) = \{P_6\}$.

The lower approximation of $P_{yes}$ is established as $B_*(P_{yes}) = \{P_1, P_5\}$ while its upper approximation is obtained as $B^*(P_{yes}) = \{P_1, P_2, P_4, P_5\}$.

The boundary set $B_{border}(P_{yes}) = \{P_2, P_4\}$ .

The membership degrees, whose sizes confirm the patients' membership in the $D_1$ = "*yes*" class, have been evaluated as

$$\mu_{D_1="yes"}(P_1) = 1, \quad \mu_{D_1="yes"}(P_2) = \frac{1}{2}, \quad \mu_{D_1="yes"}(P_3) = 0, \quad \mu_{D_1="yes"}(P_4) = \frac{1}{2},$$

$$\mu_{D_1="yes"}(P_5) = 1, \quad \mu_{D_1="yes"}(P_6) = 0.$$

We can assume that $P_1$ and $P_5$ have $D_1$ with a one hundred percent confidence, while $P_2$ and $P_4$ may suffer from $D_1$ to a certain grade. We can also notice that $P_4$ affects a status of $P_2$ negatively, and to the contrary, we can see that $P_2$ upgrades an importance of $P_4$ as a member in the $D_1$ = "*yes*"-class.

The accuracy approximation coefficient $\alpha_B(P_{yes}) = \frac{1}{2}$ does not give us a feeling of absolute trust in the choice of set $B$ as a reliable source of information in the finished classification. This configuration of symptoms is not sufficient for a reliable classification since the accuracy coefficient has a low value of 0.5.

The supplementary solutions, proposed in Chapter 4, may improve the basic diagnosis model discussed in Chapter 3. We may apply them in the patients' cases that provide us with fuzzy data difficult to interpret in order to make a reliable decision. We thus should realize that a combination of different mathematical methods could support and improve an appropriate solution that is founded on clinical symptoms.

# 5 Evaluation of Medicine Action Levels

## 5.1 Introduction

In the previous chapters, we have discussed some ways of determining the most credible diagnosis in a patient who could be identified by his set of clinical symptoms. The same symptoms are usually found in several illnesses. Therefore, it is often difficult to recognize the value of each of their deterministic yet individual characteristics all at once. After improving the diagnostic model by adding complementary solutions we are at last aware of a diagnosis of the patient. The next step would be to prescribe him medication that will lead to a cure. It is seldom possible to give the patient only one remedy to remove completely all unfavourable symptoms. In order to broaden a list of medicines that complement each other, we usually want to evaluate levels of one medicine and its impact on all of the symptoms. Preferably, we want to estimate the lowest and the highest levels of effectiveness of the medicines tested, one by one, when considering their curative powers.

We make a simple attempt of eigen fuzzy set theory applications to respond to the question concerning the possibility of deciding the degree of effectiveness on a drug that is expected to affect some of the determined symptoms. It can be concluded that a final minimal and maximal level of the drug's action, found theoretically, does not change even if the patient takes the medicine for a long time. Such a conclusion is the result of adopting the eigen fuzzy set associated with a given fuzzy relation.

The existence of the greatest eigen fuzzy set of a fuzzy relation was confirmed in the 1980's [34, 72, 73, 78]. In the latest investigations, the scientists have proved that even the least eigen fuzzy set can be generated for the given relation [4, 24, 37]. The eigen fuzzy sets have already been applied to the evaluationf of a medicine's action levels when considering the medicine influence on clinical symptoms [27, 31, 64].

The basic operation, performed in the eigen problem, is the max-min composition already introduced in Chapter 2.

## 5.2 Theoretical Assumptions of Eigen Fuzzy Problem

By studying the contents of Def. 2.11 we have approached the conception of a composition of two fuzzy relations.

Elisabeth Rakus-Andersson: *Fuzzy and Rough Techniques in Medical Diagnosis and Medication*,
StudFuzz **212**, 93–126 (2007)
www.springerlink.com

If we suppose that one of these relations is a fuzzy set, we can make the max-min composition between the relation and the set, see Section 2.5. If the result of the composition is known in advance, then we will be prepared for demonstrating a particular case of the relation composition known as the eigen fuzzy problem.

**Definition 5.1**

Assume that $X = \{x\}$ is a set of real numbers. The eigen fuzzy set of a fuzzy relation $R \subseteq X \times X$ is a set $A \subseteq X$ that satisfies the condition $A \circ R = A$.

*R* is the fuzzy relation determined as $R \subseteq X \times X$ with the membership function $\mu_R : X \times X \to [0,1]$, $\mu_R(x,x') \in [0,1]$, $x$, $x' \in X$. We prove that the eigen fuzzy set $A \subseteq X$, $\mu_A : X \to [0,1]$, $\mu_A(x) \in [0,1]$, $x \in X$, satisfying $A \circ R = A$, should exist.

Some theoretical considerations that confirm the existence of set *A* are based on the papers of Sanchez [73, 74].

We define set $A_0$ with $\mu_{A_0}(x) = a_0$ for all $x \in X$, where

$$a_0 = \min_{x' \in X}(\max_{x \in X} \mu_R(x,x')) .$$

The fuzzy connection $A_0 \circ R = A_0$ is a true equality because of

$$\mu_{A_0 \circ R}(x') = \max_x(\min(\mu_{A_0}(x), \mu_R(x,x'))) = \max_x(\min(a_0, \mu_R(x,x')))$$

$$= \min(a_0, \max_x \mu_R(x,x')) = a_0 = \mu_{A_0}(x'),\ x,\ x' \in X.$$

Hence, $A_0$ is an eigen fuzzy set of *R*.

We have shown that at least one eigen fuzzy set can be found because the equation $A_0 \circ R = A_0$ is a true statement.

The next set $A_1$ is identified by its membership function given by

$$\mu_{A_1}(x') = \max_{x \in X} \mu_R(x,x') \tag{5.1}$$

for all $x' \in X$.

The fuzzy sets, which are members of the sequence $(A_n)_n$

$$A_2 = A_1 \circ R = A_1 \circ R^1,\ A_3 = A_2 \circ R = A_1 \circ R^2, \cdots, A_{n+1} = A_n \circ R = A_1 \circ R^n, \tag{5.2}$$

exist for all integers $n > 0$.

The sets satisfy inclusions

$$A_0 \subseteq \cdots \subseteq A_{n+1} \subseteq A_n \subseteq \cdots \subseteq A_2 \subseteq A_1. \tag{5.3}$$

Before starting to prove (5.3) we will insert the definition of an inclusion $A \subseteq B$ for two fuzzy sets *A* and *B* [12, 40, 88, 95].

**Definition 5.2**

Let $A = \{(x, \mu_A(x))\}$ and $B = \{(x, \mu_B(x))\}$ be two finite fuzzy sets in $X$. We say that $A$ is a fuzzy subset of $B$ ($A \subseteq B$) if $\mu_A(x) \leq \mu_B(x)$ for every $x \in X$.

**Example 5.1**

We define $X = [0, 100]$. Let $A$ be a fuzzy set given by $\mu_A(x) = s(x, 30, 50, 70)$ and let $B$ be another fuzzy set introduced by $\mu_B(x) = s(x, 10, 50, 90)$. Since $\mu_A(x) \leq \mu_B(x)$ for all $x \in X$, as Fig. 5.1 reveals, then $A \subseteq B$.

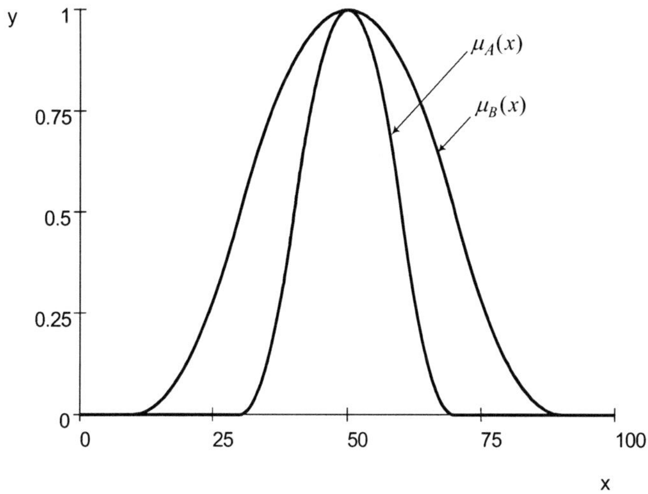


Figure 5.1: $A \subseteq B$ for $\mu_A(x) = s(x, 30, 50, 70)$ and $\mu_B(x) = s(x, 10, 50, 90)$

To confirm (5.3) we apply the mathematical induction. This method helps to prove the validity of a formula that contains a non-negative integer $n$. In order to accomplish the induction proof we follow three steps:

1. The formula should be true for $n = 0$ (or other low values of $n$).
2. We assume that the formula is valid for $n$.
3. We prove the reliability of the formula for $n + 1$ by applying the induction assumption in the proof.

Let us take $n = 0$. On the basis of the definition of $A_0$ we conclude that $A_0 \subseteq A_1$ since $\mu_{A_0}(x') = \min_{x'}(\max_{x} \mu_R(x, x')) \leq \max_{x} \mu_R(x, x') = \mu_{A_1}(x')$. We will deduce that an inclusion $A_2 \subseteq A_1$ is also true. By conveying, that $\mu_{A_2}(x') = \mu_{A_1 \circ R}(x') =$

$\max_{x \in X}(\min(\mu_{A_1}(x), \mu_R(x,x'))) \le \max_{x \in X} \mu_R(x,x') = \mu_{A_1}(x')$, for every $x' \in X$, we use Def. 5.2 to state that $A_2 \subseteq A_1$.

We should now prove that an assumption $A_n \subseteq A_{n-1}$ induces the conclusion $A_{n+1} \subseteq A_n$, $n \in N \cup \{0\}$. We start with the assumption to get an implication $A_n \subseteq A_{n-1} \to A_n \circ R \subseteq A_{n-1} \circ R \leftrightarrow A_{n+1} \subseteq A_n$, whose thesis $A_{n+1} \subseteq A_n$ is the true statement (the sign "$\leftrightarrow$" still stands for "is equivalent to").

The set $A_0$ is the eigen set of $R$. $A_1$, the other introduced set, rarely is a solution of the restriction $A_1 \circ R = A_1$. If $A_n \circ R = A_n$, for $A_n$ being a member of the sequence of sets given by (5.2), we will allege that $A_n$ is the expected greatest eigen set of the relation $R$ that differs from $A_0$. The set $A_0$ is the least set in the chain of sets in (5.2), and all sets included between $A_1$ and $A_n$ are not eigen.

Suppose that $A_0 \ne A_{n+k} = \cdots = A_{n+1} = A_n \ne \cdots \ne A_2 \ne A_1$; then the composition $A_n \circ R$ leads to $A_n \circ R = A_1 \circ R^{n-1} \circ R = A_1 \circ R^n = A_{n+1} = A_n$.

$A_n$ thus is the greatest eigen fuzzy set of $R$ provided that $A_n = A_{n+1}$. The inclusion (5.3) ensures that $A_n \subseteq A_1$. Moreover, the inclusion confirms the existence of at least one $A_n$.

The introduction of the eigen set item is sufficient for medical applications proposed in the further part of this chapter. For more mathematical details; we refer to works by Sanchez and other authors who have developed this topic [34, 72, 73, 78].

There exist three fundamental algorithms of determining GEFS (the Greatest Eigen Fuzzy Set). We prefer adopting the procedure that consists of the commands listed below.

**Algorithm 5.1**

A relation $R \subseteq X \times X$ with the membership function $\mu_R(x,x')$ is given.

1. Find the set $A_1$ identified by $\mu_{A_1}(x') = \max_{x \in X} \mu_R(x,x')$ for all $x' \in X$.
2. Set the index $n = 1$.
3. Calculate $A_{n+1} = A_n \circ R$.
4. $A_{n+1} \overset{?}{=} A_n \begin{smallmatrix} \to No \to n=n+1 \to \text{Go to step 3} \\ \to Yes \to A = A_{n+1}. \end{smallmatrix}$

We recall that membership degrees of $A_{n+1}$ are calculated as

$$\mu_{A_{n+1}}(x') = \mu_{A_n \circ R}(x') = \max_{x \in X}(\min(\mu_{A_n}(x), \mu_R(x,x'))) \tag{5.4}$$

for each $x' \in X$.

We demonstrate an action of the algorithm by selecting the greatest fuzzy set of a matrix introduced in the next example.

**Example 5.2**

We wish to find the greatest fuzzy set of a matrix

$$R = \begin{array}{c} x_1 \\ x_2 \\ x_3 \end{array} \overset{\begin{array}{ccc} x_1 & x_2 & x_3 \end{array}}{\begin{bmatrix} 0.7 & 0.5 & 0.1 \\ 0.4 & 0.6 & 0.3 \\ 0.9 & 0.8 & 0.2 \end{bmatrix}}$$

defined on $X \times X$, for $X = \{x_1, x_2, x_3\}$. The set $A_1$ has the membership degrees of $x_j$ found as the largest values in columns $j$, $j = 1, 2, 3$, and is thus determined as

$$A_1 = \overset{\begin{array}{ccc} x_1 & x_2 & x_3 \end{array}}{\begin{bmatrix} 0.9 & 0.8 & 0.3 \end{bmatrix}}.$$

For $n = 1$ we obtain

$$A_2 = A_1 \circ R = \begin{bmatrix} 0.9 & 0.8 & 0.3 \end{bmatrix} \circ \begin{bmatrix} 0.7 & 0.5 & 0.1 \\ 0.4 & 0.6 & 0.3 \\ 0.9 & 0.8 & 0.2 \end{bmatrix} = \begin{bmatrix} 0.7 & 0.6 & 0.3 \end{bmatrix}.$$

We estimate $\mu_{A_2}(x_1)$, according to the max-min composition, as the quantity $\mu_{A_2}(x_1) = \max(\min((0.9,0.7),(0.8,0.4),(0.3,0.9))) = 0.7$.

Since $A_2 \neq A_1$, we set $n = 2$ in Step 4. of Algorithm 5.1 in order to compute $A_3$ as a set

$$A_3 = A_2 \circ R = \begin{bmatrix} 0.7 & 0.6 & 0.3 \end{bmatrix} \circ \begin{bmatrix} 0.7 & 0.5 & 0.1 \\ 0.4 & 0.6 & 0.3 \\ 0.9 & 0.8 & 0.2 \end{bmatrix} = \begin{bmatrix} 0.7 & 0.6 & 0.3 \end{bmatrix}$$

that satisfies the equality $A_3 = A_2$. The set $A_3$ is accepted as the greatest eigen fuzzy set of the relation $R$ and we notice that $A_3$ holds $A_3 \subseteq A_2 \subseteq A_1$.

It can be desirable to find the smallest eigen fuzzy set of a given fuzzy relation as well. In spite of some accomplished investigations [4, 24] let us propose our own contribution as the following proof of the least eigen fuzzy set existence.

We define a new set $A_0$ with $\mu_{A_0}(x) = a_0$ for all $x \in X$, where

$a_0 = \max_{x' \in X}(\min_{x \in X} \mu_R(x, x'))$. $A_0$ is the eigen set of $R$ as it has been proved before.

The set $A_1$ also gets new membership degrees determined by

$$\mu_{A_1}(x') = \min_{x \in X} \mu_R(x, x') \tag{5.5}$$

for all $x' \in X$.

We preserve the same sequence of fuzzy sets $(A_n)_n$, $A_2 = A_1 \circ R = A_1 \circ R^1$, $A_3 = A_2 \circ R = A_1 \circ R^2, \cdots, A_{n+1} = A_n \circ R = A_1 \circ R^n$ that satisfy inclusions

$$A_1 \subseteq A_2 \subseteq \cdots \subseteq A_n \subseteq A_{n+1} \subseteq \cdots \subseteq A_0. \tag{5.6}$$

The boundary inclusion $A_1 \subseteq A_0$ in the chain is true because of $\mu_{A_0}(x') = \max_{x'}(\min_{x} \mu_R(x, x')) \geq \min_{x} \mu_R(x, x') = \mu_{A_1}(x')$.

To prove other inclusions in (5.6) we once again recall the assumptions of mathematical induction. To check if $A_1 \subseteq A_2$ we evaluate relationships among the membership degrees of both investigated sets. We make a comparison $\mu_{A_2}(x') = \mu_{A_1 \circ R}(x') = \max_{x \in X}(\min(\mu_{A_1}(x), \mu_R(x, x'))) \geq \min_{x \in X} \mu_R(x, x') = \mu_{A_1}(x')$, with respect to $x' \in X$, to get $A_2 \supseteq A_1$ according to Def. 5.2.

The last connection certainly confirms that $A_1 \subseteq A_2$ since $\mu_{A_1}(x') \leq \mu_{A_2}(x')$.

The induction assumption $A_{n-1} \subseteq A_n$ is utilized in the proof to get the conclusion $A_n \subseteq A_{n+1}$. We begin with $A_{n-1} \subseteq A_n$ to compose both sides of the inclusion with $R$ in the way: $A_{n-1} \circ R \subseteq A_n \circ R$. The last inclusion is equivalent to $A_n \subseteq A_{n+1}$.

As in the previous case the set $A_0$ is the eigen set of $R$, while $A_1$ seldom is regarded as eigen. Let us assume that $A_n$ is one of the sets listed in (5.6) and fulfils $A_n \circ R = A_n$ for $A_1 \neq A_2 \neq \cdots \neq A_n = A_{n+1} = \cdots = A_{n+k} \neq A_0$. Then $A_n$ will be the least eigen fuzzy set (LEFS) of the relation $R$ that is different from $A_0$. We notice that $A_0$ is the greatest set in the collection of sets in (5.6) and eigen as well, and we cannot find other eigen sets between $A_1$ and $A_n$, thus $A_n$ must be the least eigen set.

To evaluate the least eigen fuzzy set of $R$ we make an important change in Algorithm 5.1, namely, we state $A_1$ accordingly to the definition proposed by (5.5).

**Algorithm 5.2**

A relation $R \subseteq X \times X$ with the membership function $\mu_R(x, x')$ is given.

1. Find the set $A_1$ defined by $\mu_{A_1}(x') = \min_{x \in X} \mu_R(x, x')$ for all $x' \in X$.
2. Set the index $n = 1$.
3. Calculate $A_{n+1} = A_n \circ R$.
4. $A_{n+1} \stackrel{?}{=} A_n \begin{array}{l} \to No \to n = n+1 \to \text{Go to step 3} \\ \to Yes \to A = A_{n+1}. \end{array}$

**Example 5.3**

By returning to Ex. 5.2 we repeat the matrix

$$R = \begin{matrix} & x_1 & x_2 & x_3 \\ x_1 & 0.7 & 0.5 & 0.1 \\ x_2 & 0.4 & 0.6 & 0.3 \\ x_3 & 0.9 & 0.8 & 0.2 \end{matrix}$$

defined on $X \times X$, $X = \{x_1, x_2, x_3\}$. We then intend to calculate the entries of the least eigen fuzzy set. The membership degrees of $x_j$ in the set $A_1$ are the smallest values in columns $j$, $j = 1, 2, 3$, when applying (5.5). Hence,

$$A_1 = \begin{matrix} x_1 & x_2 & x_3 \\ [0.4 & 0.5 & 0.1] \end{matrix}.$$

For $n = 1$ we create $A_2$ as a fuzzy set

$$A_2 = A_1 \circ R = [0.4 \quad 0.5 \quad 0.1] \circ \begin{bmatrix} 0.7 & 0.5 & 0.1 \\ 0.4 & 0.6 & 0.3 \\ 0.9 & 0.8 & 0.2 \end{bmatrix} = [0.4 \quad 0.5 \quad 0.3].$$

that satisfies $A_2 \neq A_1$. We thus put $n = 2$ in Algorithm 5.2 to find $A_3$

$$A_3 = A_2 \circ R = [0.4 \quad 0.5 \quad 0.3] \circ \begin{bmatrix} 0.7 & 0.5 & 0.1 \\ 0.4 & 0.6 & 0.3 \\ 0.9 & 0.8 & 0.2 \end{bmatrix} = [0.4 \quad 0.5 \quad 0.3].$$

$A_3$ is the component of the equality $A_3 = A_2$. The set $A_3$ will be treated as the least eigen fuzzy set of the relation $R$. By the way, we check that $A_1 \subseteq A_2 \subseteq A_3$, which confirms the proper choice of the least set.

The relation $R$ keeps the given fuzzy set invariant. An occurrence in which the system (the matrix) does not produce any effect on the given input (the eigen set), apparently fits to the medical appearance when a medicine has no more effect in the curative process. If the relation is stated as "pharmacological knowledge" about some configurations of drug effectiveness created for pairs of symptoms, then an eigen set of the relation estimates, via its membership degrees, the medicine effectiveness level related to each symptom.

In the next subsection, we will suggest two definitions of fuzzy relations of the "pharmacological knowledge" type. The relations contribute in deciding the membership degrees of eigen fuzzy sets associated with them. These in turn give us a tool of determining the lowest and the highest threshold of the drug action on a collection of selected medical symptoms.

## 5.3 Eigen Sets in Medicine Effectiveness Levels

By possessing the results of examinations carried out on a group of patients with some symptoms, we can then estimate a theoretical level of effectiveness concerning medicine that is recommended to the patients belonging to the considered group. We involve the eigen problem technique for fuzzy sets to make a trial of finding the minimal and the maximal level of recovery. Although the range is stated theoretically, it ought not to change in practice during an extended period of treatment.

Let us assume that some characteristic symptoms are found in a sample of $m$ observed patients. All patients have the same symptoms. These should disappear entirely after the treatment if the drug is highly effective. Nevertheless, the symptoms can persist when the drug is not efficient enough.

Let us denote a set of symptoms by $S = \{S_1, \ldots, S_n\}$. $S_j$ is the $j^{\text{th}}$ symptom, $j = 1, \ldots, n$, and $S$ is non-fuzzy.

The estimation of the maximal level is possible by employing a fuzzy relation, created due course to the definition formulated by a sentence: "The action of the drug on the $j^{\text{th}}$ symptom is equal or stronger than on the $k^{\text{th}}$ symptom in patient, $j, k = 1, \ldots, n$". We call the relation $R_{\max}$ and we realize that $R_{\max}$ is a set of pairs $(S_j, S_k)$. The membership degree $\mu_{R_{\max}}(S_j, S_k)$, as a number from the range [0, 1], indicates the grade to which the statement defining $R_{\max}$ is true for the $j^{\text{th}}$ and the $k^{\text{th}}$ symptom [27, 31].

A comparison of the drug's influence on the considered symptoms has to be executed for each pair of the relation $R_{\max}$. Suppose that $m$ denotes a number of patients having been examined (the sample cardinality). If $b$ stands for a number of patients for whom the description of $R_{\max}$ constitutes a true sentence, then we will compute the membership degrees $\mu_{R_{\max}}(S_j, S_k)$ as

$$\mu_{R_{\max}}(S_j, S_k) = \frac{b}{m} \tag{5.7}$$

for $j, k = 1, \ldots, n$.

**Example 5.4**

As a simple example that explains a way of estimating the membership degree for two symptoms included in the same pair, we consider a group consisted of seven patients. Suppose that "–" is assigned as the lack of a symptom after the treatment and "+" designates its presence in the patient after the medication [27, 31].

To count $b$, we should consider two configuration patterns of these signs, i.e.,
"–" "–" that is interpreted as "The drug acts as strongly on $S_j$ as on $S_k$",
"–" "+" that corresponds to "The drug acts more strongly on $S_j$ than on $S_k$".

The first combination of signs signals that the examined patient is now rid of both symptoms tied to each other by the considered pair order. The second arrangement of signs explains that the patient is recovered from the first symptom while the second symptom is still prevailing after the treatment.

These configurations can be arranged as the contents of Table 5.1.

Table 5.1: Sign configurations for symptoms $S_j$, $S_k$ in $P_1$–$P_7$

| Patient | $S_j$ | $S_k$ |
|---|---|---|
| $P_1$ | – | – |
| $P_2$ | – | + |
| $P_3$ | – | + |
| $P_4$ | + | + |
| $P_5$ | – | – |
| $P_6$ | + | – |
| $P_7$ | + | + |

The membership degree of the pair ($S_j$, $S_k$) is evaluated as 0.571 (4/7) and for ($S_k$, $S_j$) as 0.429 (3/7).

The fuzzy relation $R_{\max}$ can be written down as a matrix

$$R_{\max} = \begin{matrix} & S_1 & S_2 & \cdots & S_n \\ \begin{matrix} S_1 \\ S_2 \\ \vdots \\ S_n \end{matrix} & \multicolumn{4}{l}{\begin{bmatrix} \mu_{R_{\max}}(S_1,S_1) & \mu_{R_{\max}}(S_1,S_2) & \cdots & \mu_{R_{\max}}(S_1,S_n) \\ \mu_{R_{\max}}(S_2,S_1) & \mu_{R_{\max}}(S_2,S_2) & \cdots & \mu_{R_{\max}}(S_2,S_n) \\ \vdots & \vdots & \ddots & \vdots \\ \mu_{R_{\max}}(S_n,S_1) & \mu_{R_{\max}}(S_n,S_2) & \cdots & \mu_{R_{\max}}(S_n,S_n) \end{bmatrix}} \end{matrix} . \tag{5.8}$$

We should emphasize that a diagonal entry $\mu_{R_{\max}}(S_j,S_j)$ of $R_{\max}$ has $b$ estimated as a number of "–" signs counted for $S_j$.

Next, we utilize the conception of the greatest eigen fuzzy set associated with the relation $R_{\max}$. Due to Def. 5.1 there exists the greatest fuzzy set in the universe $S$ that is associated with $R_{\max}$. The set is called $A_{\max}$, and we include it, as a crucial part, in an equation

$$A_{\max} \circ R_{\max} = A_{\max} . \tag{5.9}$$

$A_{\max}$ is a result of computations due to Algorithm 5.1, in which $A_1$ is defined by (5.1). The relation, designed in accordance with the statement: "The drug acts equally or more strongly on the $j^{\text{th}}$ symptom than on the $k^{\text{th}}$ symptom, $j$, $k = 1, \ldots, n$", has its eigen set $A_{\max}$. The set $A_{\max}$ does not change in spite of many compositions with the relation. This lack of variations leads to a conclusion that the membership degrees of $A_{\max}$ show a level: "the drug action on the considered symptoms is not stronger". $A_{\max}$ can thus be an indicator of how to estimate the maximal level to which the medicine can be effective since, evidently, $A_{\max}$ is the greatest solution of Eq. (5.9) in the sense of the largest membership degree values.

Estimation of the minimal medicine effect aims at stating another fuzzy relation $R_{\min}$ proposed as a clue: "The action of the drug on the $j^{\text{th}}$ symptom is equal or weaker than on the $k^{\text{th}}$ symptom in patient, $j, k = 1, \ldots, n$." The suggested formula of calculating membership degrees of $R_{\min}$ is similar to Eq. (5.7), but arrangements of the signs used before should be reconsidered to find $b$. We take into account the configurations:

"–" "–" that is valid if: "The drug acts as strongly on $S_j$ as on $S_k$",

"+" "–" that is approved if: "The drug acts more weakly on $S_j$ than on $S_k$".

The relation $R_{\min}$ also generates its own, this time the least, eigen fuzzy set $A_{\min}$ that constitutes the compound of an equation

$$A_{\min} \circ R_{\min} = A_{\min} \,. \tag{5.10}$$

To decide $A_{\min}$ we perform the steps of Algorithm 5.2 in which the membership function of $A_1$ is yielded by (5.5).

Since $A_{\min}$ does not change its membership degrees after the next composition with $R_{\min}$ = "The drug works equally or more weakly for the $j^{\text{th}}$ symptom in comparison to the $k^{\text{th}}$ symptom", then the membership degrees of the least eigen set, corresponding to symptoms $S_1, \ldots, S_n$, should point out the minimal effectiveness level. $A_{\min}$ is the least eigen set of $R_{\min}$, and its existential meaning can be adequate to the thesis "the action of the medicine on the considered symptoms cannot be weaker".

We treat the values of $\mu_{A_{\min}}(S_j)$ and $\mu_{A_{\max}}(S_j)$, $j = 1, \ldots, n$, as borders of this interval that limits the range of medicine effectiveness for each symptom $S_j$. Even if we obtain ranges for single symptoms, we should realize that these results are effects of the simultaneous appreciation of the medicine strength measured for pairs of symptoms when following the relations' definitions.

**Example 5.5**

The diagnosis $D$ known as a throat inflammation is recognized by the set of symptoms $S = \{S_1 =$ "*sore throat (pain)*", $S_2 =$ "*temperature*", $S_3 =$ "*inflammation state*"$\}$. The physician has prescribed *Bayer's aspirin* as a remedy that should improve the health conditions in the group of 30 patients suffering from throat inflammation.

By applying Eq. (5.7) and the sign pattern "–" "–" and "–" "+" we compute $A_{\max}$ as

$$R_{\max} = \begin{array}{c} \\ S_1 \\ S_2 \\ S_3 \end{array} \begin{array}{c} \begin{array}{ccc} S_1 & S_2 & S_3 \end{array} \\ \begin{bmatrix} 0.5 & 0.5 & 0.5 \\ 0.8 & 0.8 & 0.8 \\ 0.6 & 0.6 & 0.6 \end{bmatrix} \end{array}$$

with the corresponding greatest eigen fuzzy set decided as

$$A_{\max} = \begin{array}{c} \begin{array}{ccc} S_1 & S_2 & S_3 \end{array} \\ \begin{bmatrix} 0.8 & 0.8 & 0.8 \end{bmatrix} \end{array}.$$

Equation (5.7), in which the quantity of the associations "–" "–" and "+" "–" constitutes a basis of the $b$ value computations, results in the relation $A_{\min}$ yielded as the matrix

$$R_{\min} = \begin{array}{c} \\ S_1 \\ S_2 \\ S_3 \end{array} \begin{array}{c} \begin{array}{ccc} S_1 & S_2 & S_3 \end{array} \\ \begin{bmatrix} 0.5 & 0.8 & 0.6 \\ 0.5 & 0.8 & 0.6 \\ 0.5 & 0.8 & 0.6 \end{bmatrix} \end{array}$$

possessing the least eigen set

$$A_{\min} = \begin{array}{c} \begin{array}{ccc} S_1 & S_2 & S_3 \end{array} \\ \begin{bmatrix} 0.5 & 0.8 & 0.6 \end{bmatrix} \end{array}.$$

By interpreting the membership degrees of $A_{\min}$ and $A_{\max}$ in the percentage scale we conclude that *Bayer's aspirin* removes $S_1$ in 50%–80% and $S_2$ – in 80%. $S_3$ disappears in 60%–80% in the sample of examined patients.

By constructing the relations we consider the drug influence on pairs of symptoms to learn about the symptoms' interactions in the process of reacting on the treatment. Even if we appreciate effectiveness levels for individual symptoms, we will be aware of the complex dependency among symptoms that affects single ranges. This aspect of complexity is an advantage of fuzzy research when comparing fuzzy results to computations of statistical ranges that do not consider interactions among the examined objects.

We have engaged two different eigen sets to estimate effectiveness ranges. In spite of this, we sometimes could not find two boundaries of the range as in the case of $S_2$. In the next subsection, we will extend the procedure of deciding eigen sets by adding to them fuzzy numbers.

## 5.4 Order Operations on Fuzzy Numbers

Our next attempt to appreciate a drug level is accomplished by using another approach to eigen fuzzy sets. In contrast to the previous method presented in Section 5.3, we introduce fuzzy numbers as the membership degrees of a relation $R$ instead of real numbers belonging to the interval [0, 1].

The fuzzy number is also a fuzzy set that fulfils some particular conditions. Since we do not intend to apply fuzzy numbers defined on finite sets, we would like to quote the definition of the fuzzy number that has a continuous support [19, 20, 22, 23, 25, 36, 40, 42, 47, 95].

**Definition 5.3**

The fuzzy number $N$ is a fuzzy set of $L$-$R$ type in the real universe $Z$ if there exist two continuous reference functions $L$, $R$ and scalars $\alpha > 0$, $\beta > 0$ included in the membership function of $N$ as follows

$$\mu_N(z) = \begin{cases} L\left(\dfrac{m-z}{\alpha}\right) & \text{for} \quad m-\alpha \le z \le m, \\ R\left(\dfrac{z-m}{\beta}\right) & \text{for} \quad m \le z \le m+\beta, \end{cases} \tag{5.11}$$

$z \in Z$, where $m$, called the mean value of $N$, is a real number, and $\alpha$ and $\beta$ are called the left and right spreads, respectively. The functions $L$ and $R$ map $R^+$ in $[0,1]$. $L$ should satisfy $L(0) = 1$, $L(z) < 1$ for every $z > 0$; $L(z) > 0$ for every $z < 1$; $L(1) = 0$. The same conditions refer to $R$. Symbolically, $N$ is denoted by $N = (m_N, \alpha_N, \beta_N)$. We state a notion of the space of fuzzy numbers in the $L$-$R$ representation as $FN(LR)$. For the purpose of medical applications, we suppose that only fuzzy numbers satisfying the condition $m_N \ge 0$ belong to the space.

To be able to construct a practical version of the membership function we propose the $L(z)$ and $R(z)$ functions as [25, 63, 64]

$$L(z) = R(z) = -z + 1 \tag{5.12}$$

for $z \in Z$.

By studying (5.11) and (5.12) we realize that $N$ is such a fuzzy set whose membership function forms a triangle with the peak at the point $(m_N, 1)$. The left side of the triangle has increasing values of the membership degrees from zero to one, while the right side is as a slope that goes down to zero.

The triangles constitute the most popular shapes of membership functions assigned to fuzzy numbers.

**Example 5.6**

We perform the operations defined by (5.11) and (5.12) to find a membership function of the fuzzy number $N = (40, 2, 3)$.

We accommodate (5.11) to $m = 40$, $\alpha = 2$, $\beta = 3$. The argument $z$ in $L(z)$ is replaced by $\frac{40-z}{2}$ and in $R(z)$ – by $\frac{z-40}{3}$. We obtain a function

$$\mu_N(z) = \begin{cases} L\left(\frac{40-z}{2}\right) = 1 - \frac{40-z}{2} = \frac{z-38}{2} & \text{for} \quad 38 \le z \le 40, \\ R\left(\frac{z-40}{3}\right) = 1 - \frac{z-40}{3} = \frac{43-z}{3} & \text{for} \quad 40 \le z \le 43, \end{cases}$$

that is plotted in Fig. 5.2.

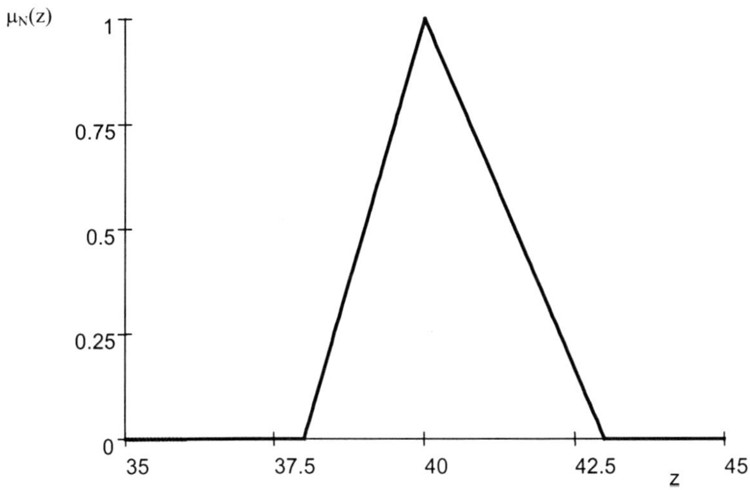


Figure 5.2: The fuzzy number $N = (40, 2, 3)$

The arithmetic over the space $FN(LR)$ is discussed in many research reports [19, 20, 22, 25, 26, 36, 40, 42, 47, 95]. In particular, order operations in $FN(LR)$ attract the scientists' attention [16, 18, 19, 20, 23, 36, 42, 47, 79, 95]. Below we discuss two sorts of order operations on fuzzy numbers in the $L$-$R$ form to select the most applicable operations and to reconsider the eigen fuzzy model.

Let us first study an approach to minimum and maximum operations proposed by Dubois and Prade [19, 20].

**Definition 5.4**

Minimum for two fuzzy numbers $N_1 = (m_{N_1}, \alpha_{N_1}, \beta_{N_1})$, $N_2 = (m_{N_2}, \alpha_{N_2}, \beta_{N_2})$ is decided to be a fuzzy number

$$\begin{aligned} &\min(N_1, N_2) = (m_{N_1}, \alpha_{N_1}, \beta_{N_1}) \\ &\text{if } m_{N_1} < m_{N_2} \text{ and } \operatorname{supp}(N_1) \cap \operatorname{supp}(N_2) = 0 \end{aligned} \tag{5.13}$$

or

$$\begin{aligned} &\min(N_1, N_2) = (\min(m_{N_1}, m_{N_2}), \max(\alpha_{N_1}, \alpha_{N_2}), \min(\beta_{N_1}, \beta_{N_2})) \\ &\text{if } m_{N_1} \neq m_{N_2} \text{ or } m_{N_1} = m_{N_2} \text{ and } \operatorname{supp}(N_1) \cap \operatorname{supp}(N_2) \neq 0\,. \end{aligned} \tag{5.14}$$

**Example 5.7**

We set $N_1 = (25, 2, 3)$ and $N_2 = (40, 1, 5)$. Since the sets $\operatorname{supp}(N_1) = [23, 28]$ and $\operatorname{supp}(N_2) = [39, 45]$ have no common elements we immediately decide that $\min(N_1, N_2) = N_1$ as pointed out in Fig. 5.3.

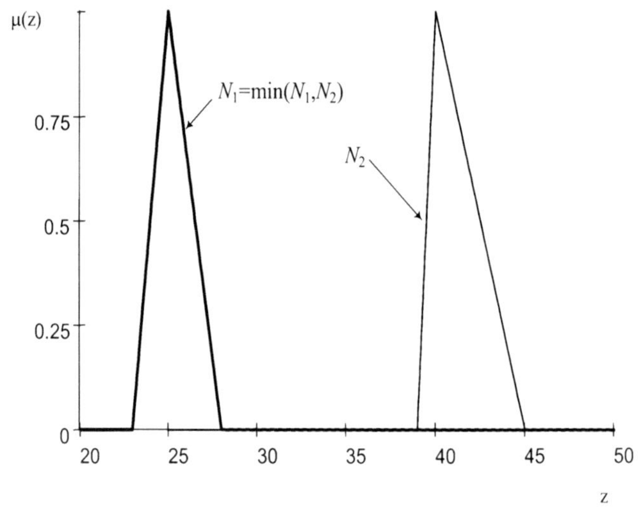


Figure 5.3: Minimum for $N_1 = (25, 2, 3)$ and $N_2 = (40, 1, 5)$ according to (5.13)

Let us explain the meaning of (5.14) by investigating data involved in the next example.

**Example 5.8**

We let $N_1 = (40, 2, 3)$ and $N_2 = (42, 1, 5)$. In accordance with (5.14), when the intersection of $\text{supp}(N_1) = [38, 43]$ and $\text{supp}(N_2) = [41, 47]$ is not the empty set, we decide $\min(N_1, N_2) = (\min(40, 42), \max(2, 1), \min(3, 5)) = (40, 2, 3)$.

The membership function of the minimal fuzzy number (40, 2, 3) has a formula

$$\mu_{(40,2,3)}(z) = \begin{cases} \dfrac{z-38}{2} & \text{for} \quad 38 \le z \le 40, \\ \dfrac{43-z}{3} & \text{for} \quad 40 \le z \le 43, \end{cases}$$

illustrated by the graph drawn in Fig. 5.4, see Ex. 5.6.

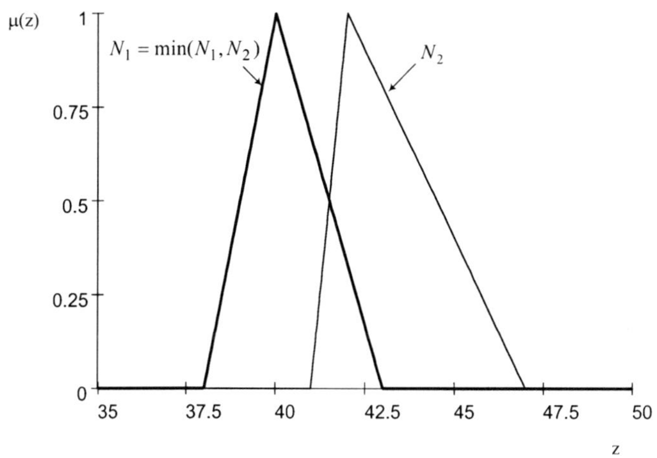


Figure 5.4: Minimum for $N_1 = (40, 2, 3)$ and $N_2 = (42, 1, 5)$ made by (5.14)

Another definition lets us determine the largest fuzzy number chosen for two numbers from the pair $(N_1, N_2)$.

**Definition 5.5**

Maximum for $N_1 = (m_{N_1}, \alpha_{N_1}, \beta_{N_1})$ and $N_2 = (m_{N_2}, \alpha_{N_2}, \beta_{N_2})$ is a fuzzy number

$$\begin{aligned} &\max(N_1, N_2) = (m_{N_1}, \alpha_{N_1}, \beta_{N_1}) \\ &\text{if } m_{N_1} > m_{N_2} \text{ and } \text{supp}(N_1) \cap \text{supp}(N_2) = 0 \end{aligned} \tag{5.15}$$

alternatively

$$\max(N_1, N_2) = (\max(m_{N_1}, m_{N_2}), \min(\alpha_{N_1}, \alpha_{N_2}), \max(\beta_{N_1}, \beta_{N_2}))$$
$$\text{if } m_{N_1} \neq m_{N_2} \text{ or } m_{N_1} = m_{N_2} \text{ and } \operatorname{supp}(N_1) \cap \operatorname{supp}(N_2) \neq 0. \tag{5.16}$$

**Example 5.9**

For two numbers from Ex. 5.7 $N_2$ is found as the rightmost element and the maximal fuzzy number in the pair ($N_1$, $N_2$) in compliance with Fig. 5.5.

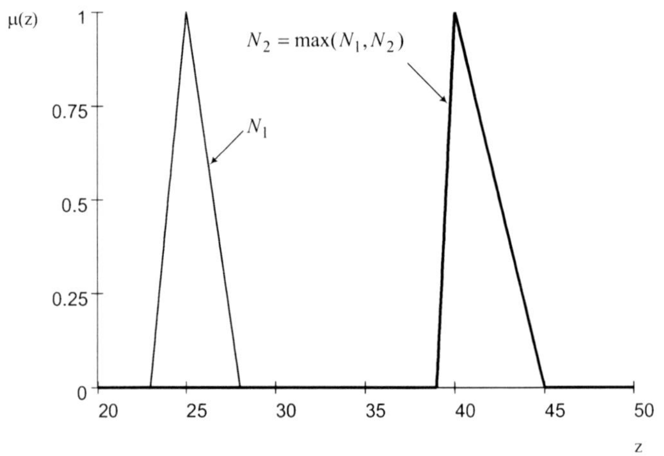


Figure 5.5: Maximum for $N_1 = (25, 2, 3)$ and $N_2 = (40, 1, 5)$ due to (5.15)

**Example 5.10**

Again we set $N_1 = (40, 2, 3)$ and $N_2 = (42, 1, 5)$. By applying (5.16) we choose $\max(N_1, N_2) = (\max(40, 42), \min(2, 1), \max(3, 5)) = (42, 1, 5)$.

The maximal fuzzy number is given by a membership function

$$\mu_{(42,1,5)}(z) = \begin{cases} L\left(\dfrac{42-z}{1}\right) = 1 - \dfrac{42-z}{1} = \dfrac{z-41}{1} & \text{for} \quad 41 \le z \le 42, \\ R\left(\dfrac{z-42}{5}\right) = 1 - \dfrac{z-42}{5} = \dfrac{47-z}{5} & \text{for} \quad 42 \le z \le 47, \end{cases}$$

sketched in Fig. 5.6.

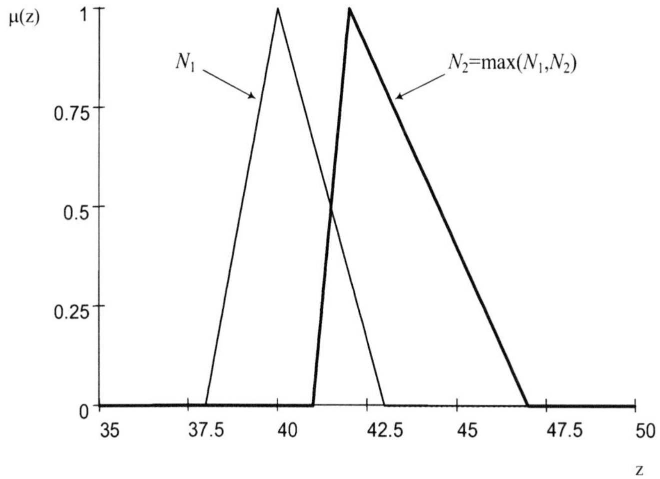


Figure 5.6: Maximum for $N_1 = (40, 2, 3)$ and $N_2 = (42, 1, 5)$ computed by (5.16)

We emphasize that the results of (5.13)–(5.14) and (5.15)–(5.16) are fuzzy numbers preserving the *L-R* representation and a triangular shape. To make some conclusions about the usability of different approaches to the concept of order among *L-R* fuzzy numbers, let us also study another attempt of defining the order operations proposed by Chih-Hui Chiu and Wen-June Wang [16].

We start with the minimum notion.

**Definition 5.6**

1) Suppose that two fuzzy numbers $N_1$ and $N_2$ given in the *L-R* representation satisfy the condition $\text{supp}(N_1) \cap \text{supp}(N_2) \neq 0$ (the supports of numbers are not disjoint). If continuous membership functions of $N_1$ and $N_2$ have one intersection point possessing the $z$-coordinate equal to $z_m$ that lies between the mean values $m_{N_1}$ and $m_{N_2}$, then

$$\mu_{\min(N_1,N_2)}(z) = \begin{cases} \max(\mu_{N_1}(z), \mu_{N_2}(z)) & \text{for} \quad z < z_m, \\ \min(\mu_{N_1}(z), \mu_{N_2}(z)) & \text{for} \quad z \geq z_m. \end{cases} \tag{5.17}$$

2) If $\text{supp}(N_1) \cap \text{supp}(N_2) = 0$ (the supports of fuzzy numbers are disjoint) then we will exploit (5.17) for any value of $z_m$ that fulfils the restriction $(z_{N_1} - z_m)(z_{N_2} - z_m) < 0$ for all $z_{N_1} \in \text{supp}(N_1)$ and all $z_{N_2} \in \text{supp}(N_2)$.

Let us first concentrate on the first part of Def. 5.6 that entails some comments.

**Example 5.11**

Once again we consider $N_1 = (40, 2, 3)$ and $N_2 = (42, 1, 5)$.

$N_1$ has the membership function expanded as (see Ex. 5.6 and Ex. 5.8)

$$\mu_{N_1}(z) = \begin{cases} \dfrac{z-38}{2} & \text{for} \quad 38 \le z < 40, \\ \dfrac{43-z}{3} & \text{for} \quad 40 \le z \le 43, \end{cases}$$

while the function of $N_2$ is expressed by (see Ex. 5.10)

$$\mu_{N_2}(z) = \begin{cases} \dfrac{z-41}{1} & \text{for} \quad 41 \le z < 42, \\ \dfrac{47-z}{5} & \text{for} \quad 42 \le z \le 47. \end{cases}$$

Both functions have an intersection point between the lines $\mu_{N_1}(z) = \dfrac{43-z}{3}$ and $\mu_{N_2}(z) = \dfrac{z-41}{1}$ that provides us with $z_m = 41.5$. Hence, we use (5.17) to get

$$\mu_{\min(N_1,N_2)}(z) = \begin{cases} \max\limits_{38 \le z \le 41.5}(\mu_{N_1}(z), \mu_{N_2}(z)) = \begin{cases} \dfrac{z-38}{2} & \text{for} \quad 38 \le z < 40, \\ \dfrac{43-z}{3} & \text{for} \quad 40 \le z \le 41.5, \end{cases} \\ \min\limits_{41.5 \le z \le 47}(\mu_{N_1}(z), \mu_{N_2}(z)) = \begin{cases} \dfrac{43-z}{3} & \text{for} \quad 41.5 \le z < 43, \\ 0 & \text{for} \quad 43 \le z \le 47, \end{cases} \end{cases}$$

$$= \mu_{N_1}(z).$$

The result of applying (5.17) is exactly the same as the effect of adopting (5.14).

To study better the action of case 2) in Def. 5.6 we should go through the next example.

**Example 5.12**

We test (5.17) related to case 2) of Def. 5.6 on $N_1 = (25, 2, 3)$ and $N_2 = (40, 1, 5)$. By returning to (5.11) and (5.12) we develop the membership function of $N_1$ as

$$\mu_{N_1}(z) = \begin{cases} L\left(\dfrac{25-z}{2}\right) = 1 - \dfrac{25-z}{2} = \dfrac{z-23}{2} & \text{for} \quad 23 \le z < 25, \\ R\left(\dfrac{z-25}{3}\right) = 1 - \dfrac{z-25}{3} = \dfrac{28-z}{3} & \text{for} \quad 25 \le z \le 28, \end{cases}$$

while the membership function of $N_2$ is equal to

$$\mu_{N_2}(z) = \begin{cases} L\left(\frac{40-z}{1}\right) = 1 - \frac{40-z}{1} = \frac{z-39}{1} & \text{for} \quad 39 \le z < 40, \\ R\left(\frac{z-40}{5}\right) = 1 - \frac{z-40}{5} = \frac{45-z}{5} & \text{for} \quad 40 \le z \le 45. \end{cases}$$

The supports [23, 28] and [39, 45] are disjoint sets. We can thus choose the value of $z_m$, say, 35 because of the condition $(z_{N_1} - 35)(z_{N_2} - 35) < 0$ that is satisfied for all $z_{N_1} \in [23,28]$ and all $z_{N_2} \in [39,45]$. By returning to (5.17) we decide minimum for $N_1$ and $N_2$ as

$$\mu_{\min(N_1,N_2)}(z) = \begin{cases} \max\limits_{23 \le z \le 35} (\mu_{N_1}(z), \mu_{N_2}(z)) = \begin{cases} \frac{z-23}{2} & \text{for} \quad 23 \le z < 25, \\ \frac{28-z}{3} & \text{for} \quad 25 \le z \le 28, \\ 0 & \text{for} \quad 28 \le z \le 35, \end{cases} \\ \min\limits_{35 \le z \le 45} (\mu_{N_1}(z), \mu_{N_2}(z)) = \{0 \qquad \text{for} \quad 35 < z \le 45, \end{cases}$$

$$= \mu_{N_1}(z).$$

Maximum for two fuzzy numbers, from the point of view presented by [16], is outlined in the following statement.

**Definition 5.7**

1) If two fuzzy numbers $N_1$ and $N_2$ obtained in the *L-R* representation have a non-empty intersection between supp($N_1$) and supp($N_2$), and if there exists one intersection point for continuous membership functions of $N_1$ and $N_2$ that has the $z$-coordinate equal to $z_m$ placed between the mean values $m_{N_1}$ and $m_{N_2}$, then

$$\mu_{\max(N_1,N_2)}(z) = \begin{cases} \min(\mu_{N_1}(z), \mu_{N_2}(z)) & \text{for} \quad z < z_m, \\ \max(\mu_{N_1}(z), \mu_{N_2}(z)) & \text{for} \quad z \ge z_m. \end{cases} \tag{5.18}$$

2) For disjoint fuzzy numbers $N_1$ and $N_2$ (supp($N_1$) ∩ supp($N_2$) = 0) we apply (5.18) for any value of $z_m$, provided that $(z_{N_1} - z_m)(z_{N_2} - z_m) < 0$ for all $z_{N_1} \in \text{supp}(N_1)$ and all $z_{N_2} \in \text{supp}(N_2)$.

**Example 5.13**

We recall $N_1 = (40, 2, 3)$ and $N_2 = (42, 1, 5)$ from Ex. 5.11. For $z_m = 41.5$ we decide $\max(N_1, N_2)$ by means of its function

$$\mu_{\max(N_1,N_2)}(z) = \begin{cases} \min\limits_{38\le z\le 41.5}(\mu_{N_1}(z), \mu_{N_2}(z)) = \begin{cases} 0 & \text{for} \quad 38 \le z < 41, \\ \dfrac{z-41}{1} & \text{for} \quad 41 \le z \le 41.5, \end{cases} \\ \max\limits_{41.5\le z\le 47}(\mu_{N_1}(z), \mu_{N_2}(z)) = \begin{cases} \dfrac{z-41}{1} & \text{for} \quad 41.5 \le z < 42, \\ \dfrac{47-z}{5} & \text{for} \quad 42 \le z \le 47, \end{cases} \end{cases}$$

$$= \mu_{N_2}(z).$$

For two non-disjoint fuzzy numbers with one intersection point between their membership functions the results of Defs 5.4, 5.6 and Defs 5.5, 5.7 are coincident. We now discuss the case of searching the minimal number for a pair $(N_1, N_2)$ that consists of fuzzy numbers intersecting each other in at least two points.

**Example 5.14**

Let $N_1 = (40, 7, 8)$ and $N_2 = (42, 3, 2)$. Let us set the numbers in (5.14) to establish $\min(N_1, N_2) = (\min(40, 42), \max(7, 3), \min(8, 2)) = (40, 7, 2)$ that preserves the triangular shape in the *L-R* form, see Fig. 5.7.

To watch effects of (5.17) we find the membership function of (40, 7, 8) as

$$\mu_{(40,7,8)}(z) = \begin{cases} \dfrac{z-33}{7} & \text{for} \quad 33 \le z < 40, \\ \dfrac{48-z}{8} & \text{for} \quad 40 \le z \le 48. \end{cases}$$

The membership function of (42, 3, 2) is computed as

$$\mu_{(42,3,2)}(z) = \begin{cases} \dfrac{z-39}{3} & \text{for} \quad 39 \le z < 42, \\ \dfrac{44-z}{2} & \text{for} \quad 42 \le z \le 44. \end{cases}$$

As $z_m$ we accept the $z$-value solving the equation $\dfrac{48-z}{8} = \dfrac{z-39}{3}$. We find $z_m =$ 41.45 and we check that it satisfies the inequality $m_{N_1} < z_m < m_{N_2}$.

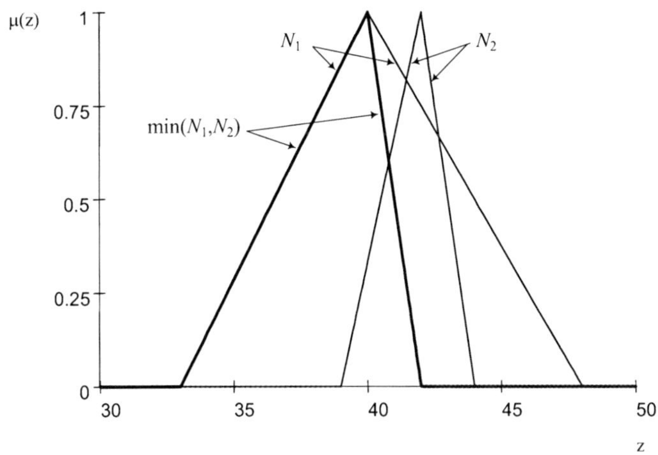


Figure 5.7: Minimum for $N_1 = (40, 7, 8)$ and $N_2 = (42, 3, 2)$ as the result of (5.14)

By expanding (5.17) we construct a function presented below and depicted in Fig. 5.8.

$$\mu_{\min(N_1,N_2)}(z) = \begin{cases} \max\limits_{33 \le z \le 41.45} (\mu_{N_1}(z), \mu_{N_2}(z)) = \begin{cases} \dfrac{z-33}{7} & \text{for} \quad 33 \le z < 40, \\ \dfrac{48-z}{8} & \text{for} \quad 40 \le z \le 41.45, \end{cases} \\ \min\limits_{41.45 \le z \le 48} (\mu_{N_1}(z), \mu_{N_2}(z)) = \begin{cases} \dfrac{48-z}{8} & \text{for} \quad 41.45 \le z < 42.67, \\ \dfrac{44-z}{2} & \text{for} \quad 42.67 \le z < 44, \\ 0 & \text{for} \quad 44 \le z \le 48, \end{cases} \end{cases}$$

The result of (5.17), found as a minimal fuzzy number for $N_1 = (40, 7, 8)$ and $N_2 = (42, 3, 2)$, does not emerge as a fuzzy number in *L-R* representation, and moreover, this minimum does not maintain the shape of a regular triangle.

The thorough analysis of properties, typical of the most popular approaches to order operations on fuzzy numbers, provides us with important hints as to the use of one alternative in further medical application. We wish to utilize these definitions of order operations on fuzzy numbers that are easy to apply, and preferably, we expect the operations to yield triangular numbers in the *L-R* form.

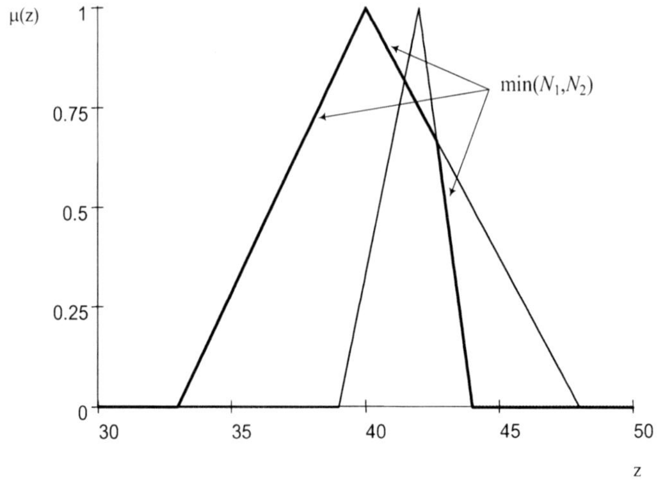


Figure 5.8: Minimum for $N_1 = (40, 7, 8)$ and $N_2 = (42, 3, 2)$ due to (5.17)

Hence, we choose operations (5.13)–(5.14) to look for the minimum and (5.15)–(5.16) to find the maximum for two fuzzy numbers in the *L-R* form. The formulas, selected above, are supposed to replace the order operations performed in algorithms that are developed to reveal eigen fuzzy sets.

## 5.5 Eigen Fuzzy Sets with Fuzzy Numbers

We use the operations on fuzzy numbers suggested by (5.13)–(5.14) and (5.15)–(5.16) to propose a new conception of the composition of a relation with a set. This time both the relation and the set have membership degrees formed as fuzzy numbers in the *L-R* form.

**Definition 5.8**

We recall that $FN(LR) = \{N : N = (m_N, \alpha_N, \beta_N)\}$.

Let $R$ be a fuzzy relation $R \subseteq X \times Y$, $X = \{x\}$, $Y = \{y\}$, with the membership function $\mu_R : X \times Y \to FN(LR)$, $\mu_R(x,y) \in FN(LR)$, $(x,y) \in X \times Y$, and let $A$ be a fuzzy set $A \subseteq X$ given by the membership function $\mu_A : X \to FN(LR)$, $\mu_A(x) \in FN(LR)$, $x \in X$.

If the membership degrees $\mu_A(x) = (m_{\mu_A(x)}, \alpha_{\mu_A(x)}, \beta_{\mu_A(x)})$ of set $A$ and the degrees $\mu_R(x,y) = (m_{\mu_R(x,y)}, \alpha_{\mu_R(x,y)}, \beta_{\mu_R(x,y)})$ of the relation $R$ are expressed by fuzzy numbers belonging to *FN*(*LR*), then we will identify the set as $B = A \circ R$ by its membership function [34, 64]

$$\mu_B(y) = (m_{\mu_B(y)}, \alpha_{\mu_B(y)}, \beta_{\mu_B(y)}) = \max_{x \in X}(\min(\mu_A(x), \mu_R(x, y)))$$
$$= \max_{x \in X}(\min((m_{\mu_A(x)}, \alpha_{\mu_A(x)}, \beta_{\mu_A(x)}), (m_{\mu_R(x,y)}, \alpha_{\mu_R(x,y)}, \beta_{\mu_R(x,y)}))) \quad (5.19)$$

for all $y \in Y$. We keep in mind that the maximum and minimum operations are performed on fuzzy numbers from *FN*(*LR*) due to (5.13)–(5.16).

**Example 5.15**

Let $X = \{10, 20, 30\}$. Set $A \subseteq X$ is a fuzzy set whose membership degrees are stated as the *L-R* fuzzy numbers, e.g., in set $Z = [0, 50]$. For instance, $A$ can be proposed as

$$A = {}^{(30,5,7)}/_{10} + {}^{(20,3,2)}/_{20} + {}^{(15,3,4)}/_{30} = \overset{\begin{matrix}10 & \quad 20 & \quad 30\end{matrix}}{\left[(30,5,7) \quad (20,3,2) \quad (15,3,4)\right]}.$$

The fuzzy relation $R \subseteq X \times X$ ($Y = X$) is constructed in the form of a $3 \times 3$ matrix. Each entry of the matrix $R$ is approved as a fuzzy number with the support constituting a subset of $Z$. We can suggest the matrix $R$ as a table

$$R = \begin{matrix} & 10 & 20 & 30 \\ 10 & (3,3,7) & (42,4,4) & (11,6,5) \\ 20 & (25,2,8) & (5,4,6) & (13,3,2) \\ 30 & (9,5,4) & (18,3,5) & (24,1,4) \end{matrix}.$$

We execute the operations suggested by (5.19), via (5.14)–(5.16) (see Ex. (5.7)–(5.10)), to get a subset of $X$ denoted by $B$ and computed as the fuzzy set

$$B = \left[(30,5,7) \quad (20,3,2) \quad (15,3,4)\right] \circ \begin{bmatrix} (3,3,7) & (42,4,4) & (11,6.5) \\ (25,2,8) & (5,4,6) & (13,3,2) \\ (9,5,4) & (18,3,5) & (24,1,4) \end{bmatrix}$$

$$= \left[(20,3,2) \quad (30,5,7) \quad (15,3,4)\right] = {}^{(20,3,2)}/_{10} + {}^{(30,5,7)}/_{20} + {}^{(15,3,4)}/_{30}$$

$B$ possesses the fuzzy numbers as its membership degrees.

**Example 5.16**

We intend to explain the difference between a type-1 (simple) fuzzy set $B_1$ and a type-2 (compound) fuzzy set $B_2$. In $B_2$ the membership degrees are given as fuzzy sets. Let us accept $B_1 = {}^{0.2}\!/_{10} + {}^{0.3}\!/_{20} + {}^{0.15}\!/_{30}$ while $B_2$ is considered as, say, the result of Ex. 5.15. We thus take $B_2 = {}^{(20,3,2)}\!/_{10} + {}^{(30,5,7)}\!/_{20} + {}^{(15,3,4)}\!/_{30}$.

The membership degrees of $B_1$ are real values from [0, 1]. Hence, set $B_1$ can be sketched in the $x$-$\mu(x)$ coordinate plane as the set of points $(x, \mu(x))$ marked by ellipses in Fig. 5.9.

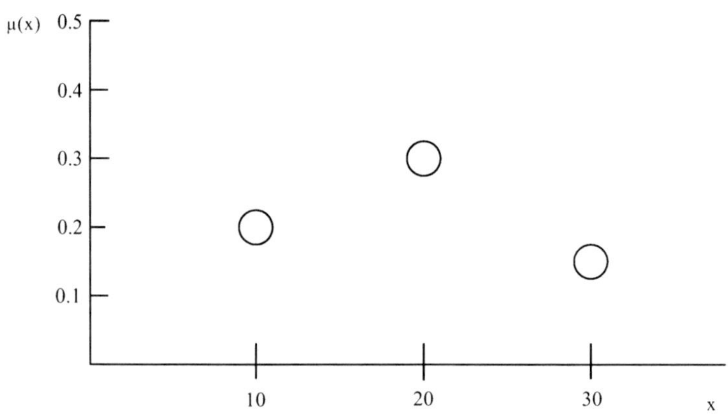


Figure 5.9: The type-1 fuzzy set $B_1 = \{(10, 0.2), (20, 0.3), (30, 0.15)\}$

The picture of $B_2$, see Fig. 5.10, is more sophisticated. We first assign supports of fuzzy numbers to the $x$-elements 10, 20, 30 belonging to $X$, and then we design the membership function for each support. The way from $x$ to $\mu(z)$ via $z$ is now three-dimensional and can be described as a path from the $x$-value to a segment along the $z$-axis and finally up along the $\mu(z)$-axis for $z \in [0, 50]$.

When set $B$ remains equal to $A$ after the max-min composition with the relation $R$ (see Def. 5.8) then we will regard $A$ as the eigen fuzzy set of relation $R$. We still assume that all membership degrees of the set and the relation appear as $L$-$R$ fuzzy numbers.

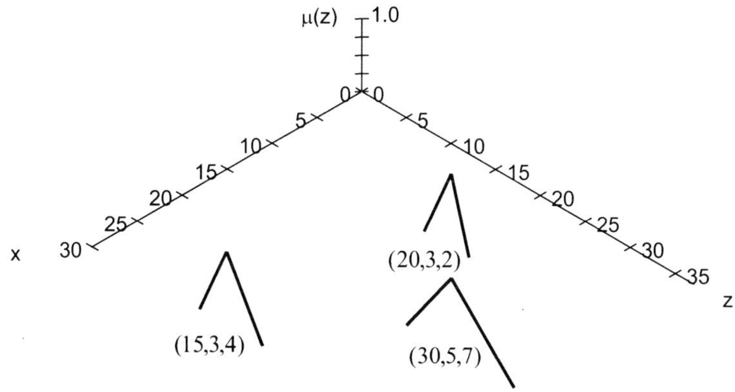


Figure 5.10: The type-2 set $B_2 = \{(10, (20, 3, 2)), (20, (30, 5, 7)), (30, (15, 3, 4))\}$

**Definition 5.9**

The eigen fuzzy set of a fuzzy relation $R \subseteq X \times X$ is a set $A \subseteq X$, $X = \{x\}$, that satisfies the condition $A \circ R = A$.

*R* is the fuzzy relation with the membership function $\mu_R : X \times X \rightarrow FN(LR)$, $\mu_R(x,x') \in FN(LR)$, *x*, *x′*∈ *X*. We should prove that the greatest eigen fuzzy set $A \subseteq X$ of relation *R*, $\mu_A : X \rightarrow FN(LR)$, $\mu_A(x) \in FN(LR)$, $x \in X$, which constitutes a crucial part of the equation $A \circ R = A$, exists [64].

Some theoretical considerations that warrant the existence of the eigen fuzzy set, possessing fuzzy numbers as the contents, are similar to the conclusions included in Subsection (5.2) and the papers of Sanchez [72, 73].

Let us first verify that the set $A_0$ with its membership function defined by $\mu_{A_0}(x) = (m_{\mu_{A_0}(x)}, \alpha_{\mu_{A_0}(x)}, \beta_{\mu_{A_0}(x)}) = (m_{N_0}, \alpha_{N_0}, \beta_{N_0})$ for all $x \in X$, where

$$(m_{N_0}, \alpha_{N_0}, \beta_{N_0}) = \min_{x' \in X} (\max_{x \in X} (m_{\mu_R(x,x')}, \alpha_{\mu_R(x,x')}, \beta_{\mu_R(x,x')})),$$

is an eigen set of *R*.

We notice that

$$\mu_{A_0 \circ R}(x') = \max_{x} (\min((m_{N_0}, \alpha_{N_0}, \beta_{N_0}), (m_{\mu_R(x,x')}, \alpha_{\mu_R(x,x')}, \beta_{\mu_R(x,x')})))$$

$$= \min((m_{N_0}, \alpha_{N_0}, \beta_{N_0}), \max_{x} (m_{\mu_R(x,x')}, \alpha_{\mu_R(x,x')}, \beta_{\mu_R(x,x')}))$$

$$= (m_{N_0}, \alpha_{N_0}, \beta_{N_0}) = \mu_{A_0}(x'),$$

since $(m_{N_0}, \alpha_{N_0}, \beta_{N_0})$ is a constant fuzzy number.

We further define the set $A_1$ by its membership function

$$\begin{aligned}\mu_{A_1}(x') &= (m_{\mu_{A_1}(x')}, \alpha_{\mu_{A_1}(x')}, \beta_{\mu_{A_1}(x')}) = \max_{x\in X} \mu_R(x,x') \\ &= \max_{x\in X}(m_{\mu_R(x,x')}, \alpha_{\mu_R(x,x')}, \beta_{\mu_R(x,x')})\end{aligned} \tag{5.20}$$

for all $x' \in X$, and we introduce the sequence $(A_n)_n$ of the type-2 fuzzy sets (the sets whose membership degrees are determined by other fuzzy sets – in this case – fuzzy numbers)

$$A_2 = A_1 \circ R = A_1 \circ R^1,\ A_3 = A_2 \circ R = A_1 \circ R^2, \cdots, A_{n+1} = A_n \circ R = A_1 \circ R^n \tag{5.21}$$

for all integers $n > 1$.

We conclude that

$$A_0 \subseteq \cdots \subseteq A_{n+1} \subseteq A_n \subseteq \cdots \subseteq A_2 \subseteq A_1 , \tag{5.22}$$

that can be compared to (5.3).

We prove the inclusions (5.22) in the same manner as the inclusions (5.3) but all the operations assisting the proofs are performed with respect to fuzzy numbers from *FN*(*LR*).

The set $A_0$ always is the eigen set of $R$, while $A_1$ sometimes is regarded as an eigen set of the considered relation. When $A_n \circ R = A_n$ for $A_n$ from the collection (5.21) then $A_n$ will be the greatest eigen set of the relation $R$, and $A_n$ seldom equals $A_0$. To put this assertion to the test we repeat this method of concluding that was already accomplished in section 5.2, but we remember that fuzzy numbers replace membership degrees in all developments involving fuzzy sets and fuzzy relations.

To find the greatest eigen set $A = A_n$ of the fuzzy relation $R$ we access Algorithm 5.1 in which we execute the operations on fuzzy numbers in accord with (5.19). As the minimum and maximum operations, we exploit (5.13)–(5.16), which warrant that the results will be obtained as numbers in the *L-R* forms. The *L-R* forms in turn facilitate the interpretation of number membership functions.

The eigen value model producing eigen sets with fuzzy numbers as the membership degrees is essential in the fitness procedure when appreciating an upper threshold of the drug action. The supports of fuzzy numbers are supposed to indicate effectiveness levels of the medicine that should bring some relief to a patient.

## 5.6 The *L-R* Fuzzy Numbers as Drug Efficiency Intervals

To obtain levels of drug efficiency that are bounded by a lower and an upper limit, we make a new attempt of solving the problem of appreciating the effectiveness level of a medicine when using it against the symptoms typical of an illness. We introduce a fuzzy relation with elements equal to fuzzy numbers in the *L-R* representation to describe some connections among the symptoms. The fuzzy numbers that appear in the relation replace the verbal expressions decided by physicians in accordance with the definition of the relation.

The fuzzy relation discussed in Subsection 2.5 is a counterpart of the fuzzy relation filled with fuzzy numbers. The latter produces an eigen fuzzy set whose membership degrees also are structured as fuzzy numbers. These, via their supports, appreciate the levels of drug influence on clinical symptoms [64].

Assume that a certain disease is characterized by some typical symptoms placed within the set of symptoms $S = \{S_1, \cdots, S_n\}$. We try to appreciate the influence level of the drug on each symptom by researching an eigen fuzzy set associated with the fuzzy relation $R \subseteq S \circ S$. We believe in the physicians' experience and therefore we believe that the essential relief concerning one symptom, e.g., sharp ache, improves the patient's mood and physical condition even if other symptoms still are present. We agree with this observation of the patients' reaction on the treatment, and as an expression of our belief, we define the relation $R$ by $R$ = "the cumulated effectiveness of the drug action for $S_i$ and $S_j$, $i, j = 1, \ldots, n$".

Let us state a content of the list with verbal descriptions of the effectiveness in accordance with the physician's advice. The list containing the grades of growing effectiveness is proposed to be $L$ = {$N_0$ = "*none*", $N_1$ = "*almost none*", $N_2$ = "*very little*", $N_3$ = "*little*", $N_4$ = "*rather little*", $N_5$ = "*medium*", $N_6$ = "*rather large*", $N_7$ = "*large*", $N_8$ = "*very large*", $N_9$ = "*almost complete*", $N_{10}$ = "*complete*"}.

In order to replace words by fuzzy numbers in the *L-R* form we utilize (5.12) and construct the membership functions of $N_k$, $k = 0, 1, 2, \ldots, 10$, as

$$\mu_{N_k}(z) = \begin{cases} L\left(\dfrac{10\cdot k - z}{10}\right) = \dfrac{z - 10\cdot k + 10}{10} & \text{for} \quad 10\cdot k - 10 \le z < 10\cdot k, \\ R\left(\dfrac{z - 10\cdot k}{10}\right) = \dfrac{10\cdot k + 10 - z}{10} & \text{for} \quad 10\cdot k \le z \le 10\cdot k + 10. \end{cases} \tag{5.23}$$

Hence

$$N_k = (10\cdot k, 10, 10)\,. \tag{5.24}$$

We are enabled to derive Eqs (5.23) in another manner as well. In similarity with Examples 3.9–3.11 we can arrange three atomic effectiveness descriptions such as "*seldom*", "*medium*" and "*large*" to get the rest of formulations by adding hedges. Later, the specified values of the parameter $\delta$ (see Subsection 3.4.1) let us model shapes of all membership functions assigned to the effectiveness terms.

**Example 5.17**

The overview of different effectiveness designs is available in Fig. 5.11. We assume that an adequate theoretical reference set for all terms describing effectiveness is chosen as $Z = [0, 100]$. This even corresponds to the percentage scale 0%–100%. Let us extend the interval to $[-10, 110]$ to make space for all supports of the fuzzy numbers associated with the effectiveness. The numbers are placed along the $z$-axis that constitutes their common domain.

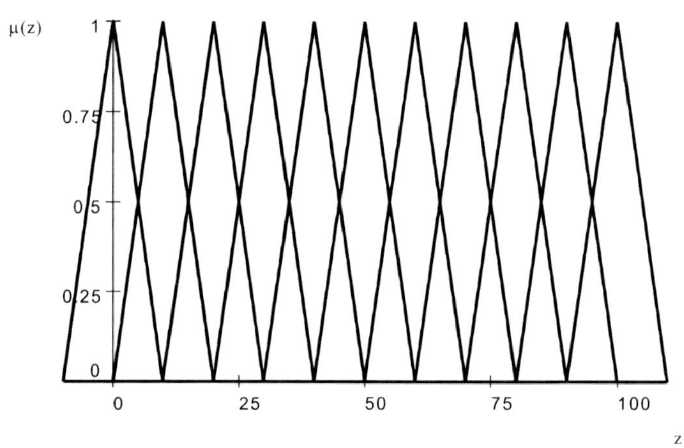


Figure 5.11: Terms of drug effectiveness expressed as fuzzy numbers

For instance, we set the value of $k = 3$ in (5.23) and involve (5.12) when we want to evaluate the membership function of "*little*" = $N_3$. The structure "*little*" = $N_3 = (30,10,10)$ has a membership function derived as

$$\mu_{N_3}(z) = \begin{cases} L\left(\dfrac{10\cdot 3 - z}{10}\right) = -\dfrac{10\cdot 3 - z}{10} + 1 = \dfrac{z-20}{10} & \text{for} \quad 20 \le z < 30, \\ R\left(\dfrac{z - 10\cdot 3}{10}\right) = -\dfrac{z-10\cdot 3}{10} + 1 = \dfrac{40-z}{10} & \text{for} \quad 30 \le z \le 40. \end{cases}$$

Denote the set of $N_0, \ldots, N_{10}$ by $E=\{N_k\}$, $k = 0, 1, \ldots, 10$. The supports of the fuzzy numbers $N_k$ are the subsets of the set $[-10,110]$ (the technical extension of $[0, 100]$ that is the best reference set used in medicine). The spreads $\alpha = \beta = 10$ are modelled after the consultation with the physicians who have advised these numbers as proper for the considered problem.

After determining some relationship between the verbal expressions graduating the effectiveness and the fuzzy numbers suggested by (5.23), we create the contents of the relation *R*. The physician assigns the semantic structure describing the effectiveness of a tested medicine to the single symptom $S_i$, $i = 1, \ldots, n$. The fuzzy number $N_k$, $k = 0, \ldots, 10$ substitutes this word afterwards. Nevertheless, we realize that we should propose a connective operator for fuzzy numbers representing the pairs of symptoms with regard to the definition of *R*.

The values of "effectiveness $(S_i) = N_{i_k}$" and "effectiveness $(S_j) = N_{j_k}$", describing the medicine curative power in the case of the symptoms $S_i$, $S_j$, $k = 0, 1, \ldots, 10$, $N_{i_k}, N_{j_k} \in E$, constitute crucial factors of the membership degree $\mu_R(S_i, S_j)$ fixed by a formula [64]

$$\begin{aligned}\mu_R(S_i,S_j) &= \frac{N_{i_k}+N_{j_k}}{2} = \frac{(m_{N_{ik}},\alpha_{N_{ik}},\beta_{N_{ik}})+(m_{N_{jk}},\alpha_{N_{jk}},\beta_{N_{jk}})}{2} \\ &= \left(\frac{m_{N_{ik}}+m_{N_{jk}}}{2}, \frac{\alpha_{N_{ik}}+\alpha_{N_{jk}}}{2}, \frac{\beta_{N_{ik}}+\beta_{N_{jk}}}{2}\right)\end{aligned} \tag{5.25}$$

for $i, j = 1, \ldots, n$.

The aggregation operation for two fuzzy numbers suggested in (5.25) is based on the mean values that sometimes are the items of critical remarks. In spite of them, experienced physicians recommend the mean operations in medicine to avoid accepting too sharp results being effects of maximum and minimum operators. We even know that OWA aggregation operator techniques based on mean values [46, 81, 83, 85], already discussed in Subsection 4.2, have acquired a high preference in different applications.

**Example 5.18**

The mean $\frac{m_{N_{ik}}+m_{N_{jk}}}{2}$ is the OWA operation for $a_0 = 0$, $a_1 = a_2 = \frac{1}{2}$ and can be expanded in the sum (5.25) as $\frac{1}{2}\min\left(m_{N_{ik}}, m_{N_{jk}}\right) + \frac{1}{2}\max\left(\min\left(m_{N_{jk}}\right), \min\left(m_{N_{ik}}\right)\right)$ accordingly to Def. 4.1.

If $m_{N_{ik}} = 40$ and $m_{N_{jk}} = 30$ then $\frac{1}{2}\min(40,30) + \frac{1}{2}\max(\min(30), \min(40)) = \frac{30}{2} + \frac{40}{2} = 35$.

The functional significance of Def. 4.1 is authorized by the results obtained in Ex. 5.18. We should now be totally convinced that the operation of computing an arithmetic mean is classified as a modern OWA operator and there is nothing wrong in its adaptation.

If some symptoms are more important than others in the clinical picture of the disease, then a weighted aggregation operation ought to be used. We define a simple and intuitive scale of weights as the set, e.g., $H = \{h_1, h_2, h_3, h_4\} = \{1,2,3,4\}$, where the value of 4 is reserved for symptom $S_i$ revealing the greatest importance in the observed disease. By *importance* we mean the harmful impact of a symptom on the patient's state. Let us estimate a membership grade $\mu_R(S_i, S_j)$ of ($S_i$, $S_j$) as

$$\begin{aligned}\mu_R(S_i,S_j) &= \frac{h_{i_l}N_{i_k} + h_{j_l}N_{j_k}}{h_{i_l}+h_{j_l}} = \frac{h_{i_l}(m_{N_{ik}}, \alpha_{N_{ik}}, \beta_{N_{ik}}) + h_{j_l}(m_{N_{jk}}, \alpha_{N_{jk}}, \beta_{N_{jk}})}{h_{i_l}+h_{j_l}} \\ &= \left(\frac{h_{i_l}m_{N_{ik}} + h_{j_l}m_{N_{jk}}}{h_{i_l}+h_{j_l}}, \frac{h_{i_l}\alpha_{N_{ik}} + h_{j_l}\alpha_{N_{jk}}}{h_{i_l}+h_{j_l}}, \frac{h_{i_l}\beta_{N_{ik}} + h_{j_l}\beta_{N_{jk}}}{h_{i_l}+h_{j_l}}\right)\end{aligned} \tag{5.26}$$

for $h_{i_l}, h_{j_l} \in H, N_{i_k}, N_{j_k} \in E$, $i, j = 1, \ldots, n$, $k = 0, 1, \ldots, 10$, $l = 1,2,3,4$. The proposed weights are related to the symptoms when the importance of the symptoms should be emphasized.

If all weights are equal to 1 it will mean no important difference among the symptoms, and consequently we return to (5.25).

**Example 5.19**

Even the operations defined by (5.26) belong to the OWA category operators. For the mean value of the fuzzy number (5.26) we consider two cases:

1) If $m_{N_{ik}} < m_{N_{jk}}$ then, for $a_0 = 0$, $a_1 = \dfrac{h_{i_l}}{h_{i_l}+h_{j_l}}$ and $a_2 = \dfrac{h_{j_l}}{h_{i_l}+h_{j_l}}$ we create

$$\frac{h_{i_l}m_{N_{ik}} + h_{j_l}m_{N_{jk}}}{h_{i_l}+h_{j_l}} = \frac{h_{i_l}}{h_{i_l}+h_{j_l}}\min(m_{N_{ik}}, m_{N_{jk}}) + \frac{h_{j_l}}{h_{i_l}+h_{j_l}}\max(m_{N_{ik}}, m_{N_{jk}}).$$

When we set, e.g., $m_{N_{ik}} = 30$, $m_{N_{jk}} = 50$, $h_{i_l} = 3, h_{j_l} = 4$ then we will make a calculus $\dfrac{3\cdot 30 + 4\cdot 50}{3+4} = \dfrac{3}{3+4}\min(30,50) + \dfrac{4}{3+4}\max(30,50)$, see (5.26).

2) For $m_{N_{ik}} > m_{N_{jk}}$ we put $a_0 = 0$, $a_1 = \dfrac{h_{j_l}}{h_{i_l}+h_{j_l}}$ and $a_2 = \dfrac{h_{i_l}}{h_{i_l}+h_{j_l}}$ in the mean value of (5.26). We compute

$$\frac{h_{i_l}m_{N_{ik}} + h_{j_l}m_{N_{jk}}}{h_{i_l}+h_{j_l}} = \frac{h_{j_l}}{h_{i_l}+h_{j_l}}\min(m_{N_{ik}}, m_{N_{jk}}) + \frac{h_{i_l}}{h_{i_l}+h_{j_l}}\max(m_{N_{ik}}, m_{N_{jk}}).$$

If , for example, $m_{N_{ik}} = 50$, $m_{N_{jk}} = 30$, $h_{i_l} = 3, h_{j_l} = 4$, then we will prove

$$\frac{3 \cdot 50 + 4 \cdot 30}{3+4} = \frac{4}{3+4}\min(30,50) + \frac{3}{3+4}\max(30,50) .$$

The relation $R$ expresses the synchronized effectiveness of the drug action for every pair of symptoms. $R$ has its eigen fuzzy set $A$ that does not change after the next composition with it. The support of $A$ consists of the elements of $S$, and the membership grades $\mu_A(S_j)$ of $S_j$, $j = 1, \ldots, n$, belonging to $A$ are fuzzy numbers in the *L-R* representation. Furthermore, the supports of the numbers can be interpreted as the levels of medicinal action for the examined symptoms one by one.

Set $A$, fulfilling $A \circ R = A$, is represented by the following connection derived for the membership functions, see (5.19)

$$\mu_{A \circ R}(S_j) = \max_{S_i \in S}(\min(\mu_A(S_i), \mu_R(S_i, S_j))) = \mu_A(S_j) = (m_{\mu_A(S_j)}, \alpha_{\mu_A(S_j)}, \beta_{\mu_A(S_j)}),$$
$$\mu_A(S_i),\ \mu_A(S_j), \mu_R(S_i, S_j) \in FN(LR), \tag{5.27}$$

in which the maximum and minimum operations are performed due to (5.13)–(5.16) for $i, j = 1, \ldots, n$ .

Let us designate $\mu_A(S_j) = (m_{\mu_A(S_j)}, \alpha_{\mu_A(S_j)}, \beta_{\mu_A(S_j)})$ as $A(S_j)$ in the next step of investigations.

Even if the levels concern single symptoms, we shall remember that the positive reaction after the treatment, assigned to one symptom, also affects the ranges of other symptoms. The levels, established by means of the eigen set, do not change in spite of the extended curative period.

**Example 5.20**

We intend to test the designed model on clinical data from Ex. 5.5 that we have already been acquainted with.

By giving the patients *Bayer's aspirin* we cure the inflammation of the throat. Patients who suffer from it are often troubled with selected symptoms; $S_1$ = "*sore throat (pain)*", $S_2$ = "*temperature*", $S_3$ = "*inflammation state*". Due to the physician's opinion the approximate effectiveness of the drug has been decided as "m" = "*medium*" for $S_1$, "vlg" = "*very large*" for $S_2$ and "lg" = "*large*" in the case of $S_3$. The fuzzy relation $R$ = "the cumulated effectiveness of the drug action for $S_i$ and $S_j$, $i, j = 1, 2, 3$" is then expressed by the table

$$R = \begin{array}{c} \\ S_1 \\ S_2 \\ S_3 \end{array}\begin{array}{c} \begin{array}{ccc} S_1 & S_2 & S_3 \end{array} \\ \begin{bmatrix} \text{"m"} & \text{"m" and "vlg"} & \text{"m" and "lg"} \\ \text{"vlg" and "m"} & \text{"vlg"} & \text{"vlg" and "lg"} \\ \text{"lg" and "m"} & \text{"lg" and vlg"} & \text{"lg"} \end{bmatrix} \end{array}.$$

After assigning the weights 4, 2 and 3 to $S_1$, $S_2$ and $S_3$ respectively, we form in accordance with (5.24) and (5.26) the table

$$R = \begin{bmatrix} \frac{4(50,10,10)}{4} & \frac{4(50,10,10)+2(80,10,10)}{4+2} & \frac{4(50,10,10)+3(70,10,10)}{4+3} \\ \frac{2(80,10,10)+4(50,10,10)}{2+4} & \frac{2(80,10,10)}{2} & \frac{2(80,10,10)+3(70,10,10)}{2+3} \\ \frac{3(70,10,10)+4(50,10,10)}{3+4} & \frac{3(70,10,10)+2(80,10,10)}{3+2} & \frac{3(70,10,10)}{3} \end{bmatrix}$$

as a counterpart of the linguistically defined relation $R$. We compute the entries of $R$ to get it in the final version

$$R = \begin{bmatrix} (50,10,10) & (60,10,10) & (59,10,10) \\ (60,10,10) & (80,10,10) & (74,10,10) \\ (59,10,10) & (74,10,10) & (70,10,10) \end{bmatrix}.$$

To determine the corresponding greatest eigen fuzzy set $A$ we exploit the steps of Algorithm 5.1 as follows.

1. $A_1$ is decided as a type-2 fuzzy set

$$A_1 = \begin{array}{c} \begin{array}{ccc} S_1 & S_2 & S_3 \end{array} \\ [(60,10,10) \quad (80,10,10) \quad (74,10,10)] \end{array}.$$

2) The action of (5.13)–(5.16) leads to the first composition of $A_1$ with $R$ and results in

$$A_2 = [(60,10,10) \quad (80,10,10) \quad (74,10,10)] \circ \begin{bmatrix} (50,10,10) & (60,10,10) & (59,10,10) \\ (60,10,10) & (80,10,10) & (74,10,10) \\ (59,10,10) & (74,10,10) & (70,10,10) \end{bmatrix}$$
$$= [(60,10,10) \quad (80,10,10) \quad (74,10,10)].$$

3) Since $A_2 = A_1$ we accept $A = A_2$.

By coming back to the formula $L(z) = R(z) = -z + 1$ we finally determine the levels of *Bayer's aspirin* curative effect as supports of the fuzzy numbers $A(S_1)$, $A(S_2)$ and $A(S_3)$, specified by membership functions

$$\mu_{A(S_1)}(z) = \begin{cases} \dfrac{z-50}{10} & \text{for} \quad 50 \le z < 60, \\ \dfrac{70-z}{10} & \text{for} \quad 60 \le z \le 70, \end{cases}$$

$$\mu_{A(S_2)}(z) = \begin{cases} \dfrac{z-70}{10} & \text{for} \quad 70 \le z < 80, \\ \dfrac{90-z}{10} & \text{for} \quad 80 \le z \le 90, \end{cases}$$

and

$$\mu_{A(S_3)}(z) = \begin{cases} \dfrac{z-64}{10} & \text{for} \quad 64 \le z < 74, \\ \dfrac{84-z}{10} & \text{for} \quad 74 \le z \le 84.. \end{cases}$$

The membership functions of $A(S_1)$, $A(S_2)$ and $A(S_3)$ are drawn in Fig. 5.12.

The results can be interpretable in the percentage scale, for the supports of fuzzy numbers are subsets of the standard population [0, 100]. We take into consideration the most important parts of the number supports associated with the membership grades greater than, say, 0.5. Summing up, we make a trial of approximating the curative effect of *Bayer's aspirin* in 55%–65% for $S_1$, 75%85% for $S_2$ and 69%–79% with respect to $S_3$.

Let us emphasize some advantages of the application of the eigen fuzzy model with fuzzy numbers to an appreciation of the drug level as follows.

Even if the fuzzy relation has the elements equal to fuzzy numbers, the eigen fuzzy set associated with the relation will exist. The supports of fuzzy numbers obtained in the eigen fuzzy set yield the expected levels of drug action for every distinct symptom.

The levels are the most optimistic prognoses of drug action since the given eigen fuzzy set is greatest. Moreover, the effects of common medicine action in regard to pairs of symptoms positively influence the range of single levels.

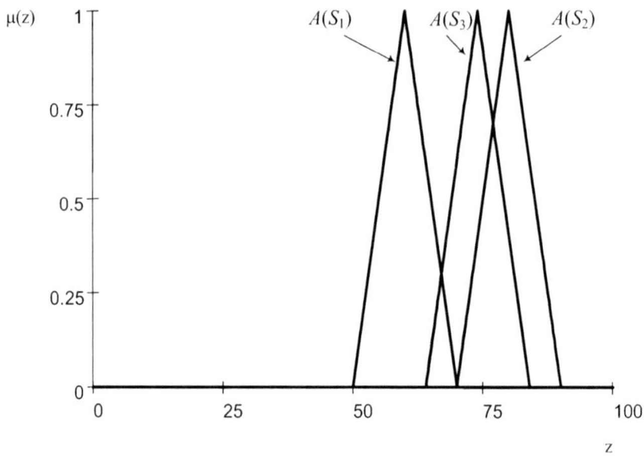


Figure 5.12: Fuzzy numbers $A(S_1)$, $A(S_2)$, $A(S_3)$ of the eigen set $A$ of the relation $R$

Even the importance of symptoms in a disease also affects the appreciation of levels. The results do not depend on any sample size that can be unstable, but they are based on the stabile expressions formulated by experienced physicians.

At last, the results should satisfy the expectations of medicine manufacturers who wish to recommend the most efficacious, curative remedy.

We have been concentrating our attention on the estimation of one-drug levels concerning several symptoms. In the next chapter, we maintain the same collection of symptoms but we make some different approaches. We will attempt the selection of the best medicine from a sample of remedies recommended in a certain disease.

# 6 The Choice of Optimal Medicines

## 6.1 Introduction

We have already used many auxiliary methods coming from fuzzy set theory to make attempts at solutions in such medical tasks as diagnosing or appreciation of drug efficiency. In Chapter 5 we have tested eigen fuzzy set techniques to appreciate the optimal levels of one drug action in the case of several symptoms characteristic of a disease.

We often experience that there can occur such a pathologic process in which the symptoms do not disappear after the treatment when using only one medicine. The medication can improve too high or too low of a level of the quantitative symptom, but the symptom still indicates the presence of the disease. We sometimes have some problems in making a choice of this medicine, which acts best; because it can happen that most drugs influence the same symptoms while they do not improve the others.

By employing different fuzzy decision-making models, we try to make it easier to find such a drug that affects most of the symptoms in the highest degree. We also want to discuss the task of selecting the best possible medicine within the circumstances provided when some decision-makers have different opinions about the priority of tested drugs.

In fuzzy decision making models, often applied to technical solutions like in [33], we also use non-fuzzy sets. It is remarkable to observe how the assumptions of fuzzy set theory link crisp sets to imprecise collections of elements to obtain a harmonic mixture of decisive information.

Some readers may still experience the advantage of translating average words originating from "spoken" languages into numbers (we have already discussed the problem in Chapter 3). This emphasizes the richness of applications offered by processes of numerical fuzzifying of some appearances that cannot be strictly defined.

## 6.2 Fuzzy Utilities in Decision-Making Models

Let us introduce the notions of a space of states-results $X = \{x_1, x_2, ..., x_m\}$ and a decision space $A = \{a_1, a_2, ..., a_n\}$. The mentioned universes of discourse constitute the main data basis in Jain's decision-making model.

Elisabeth Rakus-Andersson: *Fuzzy and Rough Techniques in Medical Diagnosis and Medication*, StudFuzz **212**, 127–154 (2007)
www.springerlink.com

### 6.2.1 Jain's Utility Matrix as the *Drug – Symptom* Table

If a rational decision maker makes a decision $a_i \in A$, $i = 1, 2, \ldots, n$, concerning states-results $x_j \in X$, $j = 1, 2, \ldots, m$, then the problem is reduced to the consideration of the ordered triplet $(X, A, U)$, where $X$ is a set of states-results, $A$ – a set of decisions and $U$ – the utility matrix [38, 39, 40]

$$U = \begin{bmatrix} U_{11} & U_{12} & \cdots & U_{1m} \\ U_{21} & U_{22} & \cdots & U_{2m} \\ \vdots & & \ddots & \vdots \\ U_{n1} & U_{n2} & \cdots & U_{nm} \end{bmatrix} \tag{6.1}$$

in which each element $U_{ij}$, $i = 1, 2, \ldots, n$, $j = 1, 2, \ldots, m$, is a fuzzy set defining the fuzzy utility following from the decision $a_i$ with the result $x_j$.

Assume now that the state-result is not exactly known, but as a fuzzy set $S \subseteq X$ given in the form

$$S = \mu_S(x_1)/x_1 + \mu_S(x_2)/x_2 + \cdots + \mu_S(x_m)/x_m \,. \tag{6.2}$$

A decision method thus concerns such fuzzy decision situation in which both the knowledge about the state and the utilities are fuzzy. To solve the decision problem under circumstances that are given above, means to find the best decision $a_i$ influenced by all constraints.

The theoretical model with the triplet $(X, A, U)$ and the fuzzy set of states $S$, thus very shortly sketched, can find its practical application in the processes of choosing an optimal drug. If a given disease is recognized by the symptoms accompanying it, then we, by giving a medicine, try to liquidate these symptoms or at least try to reduce their unfavorable influence upon the patient's health. Not all symptoms retreat after the cure has been carried out. Sometimes, one can only soothe their negative effects by, for example, the lowering of an excessive level of the indicator, the relief of pain, and the like, but cannot ascertain that the patient is fully free from them. The problem of choosing an optimal drug (decision), which soothes the symptoms or has some power to eliminate them in full, corresponds to the theoretical assumptions presented above [59, 60, 62].

In order to show the algorithm for finding such a decision let us consider a model with $n$ drugs $a_1, a_2, \ldots, a_n \in A$. On the basis of the physician's decision, the drugs are prescribed to the patient (thus may be treated as decisions $a_1, a_2, \ldots, a_n$) with a view to have an effect on $m$ symptoms $x_1, x_2, \ldots, x_m \in X$ representing certain states characteristic of the given disease. We actually rename the symptoms as $x_j$ instead for $S_j$ as we used in Chapters 3–5 to agree with some symbolic terms assigned to states-results being parts of fuzzy decision-making models. To simplify the symbols let us further assume that each symptom $x_j \in X$, where $X$ is a space of symptoms (states), is understood as the result of the treatment of the symptom after the cure with the drugs $a_1, a_2, ..., a_n$ has been carried out. On the basis of earlier experiments the physician knows how to define in words the curative drug efficiency in the case of considered symptoms. In accordance with his advice, we suggest a list of terms, already known from Section 5.6 that introduces a linguistic variable named "the curative drug effectiveness regarding a symptom" = {$R_1$ ="*none*", $R_2$ = "*almost none*", $R_3$ = "*very little*", $R_4$ = "*little*", $R_5$ = "*rather little*", $R_6$ = "*medium*", $R_7$ = "*rather large*", $R_8$ = "*large*", $R_9$ = "*very large*", $R_{10}$ = "*almost complete*", $R_{11}$ = "*complete*"}. Each notion from this list of terms is the name of a fuzzy set. Assume that all sets are defined in the space $Z = [0,100]$, see Ex. 5.17, which is suitable as a reference set to measure a number of patients who have been affected by a medicine in the grade corresponding to each name. We use this technique of building a list of expressions for the third time. Each time we change the forms of constraints to demonstrate how many options in the creation of membership functions are allowable.

To avoid further complicated computations we suggest membership functions of the fuzzy sets from the list, called "the curative drug effectiveness regarding a symptom", as simple linear functions [2, 59, 60, 62]

$$L(z,\alpha,\beta) = \begin{cases} 0 & \text{for } z \le \alpha, \\ \dfrac{z-\alpha}{\beta-\alpha} & \text{for } \alpha < z \le \beta, \\ 1 & \text{for } z > \beta, \end{cases} \tag{6.3}$$

and

$$\pi(z,\alpha,\gamma,\beta) = \begin{cases} 0 & \text{for } z \le \alpha, \\ L(z,\alpha,\gamma) & \text{for } \alpha < z \le \gamma, \\ 1 - L(z,\gamma,\beta) & \text{for } \gamma < z \le \beta, \\ 0 & \text{for } z > \beta, \end{cases} \tag{6.4}$$

where $z$ is an independent variable belonging to [0, 100] and $\alpha$, $\beta$, $\gamma$ are some parameters.

Let us define

$$\mu_{R_k}(z) = \begin{cases} 1 - L(z,\alpha_k,\beta_k) & \text{for } k = 1,2,3,4,5, \\ L(z,\alpha_k,\beta_k) & \text{for } k = 7,8,9,10,11, \end{cases} \tag{6.5}$$

and

$$\mu_{R_6}(z) = \pi(z, \alpha_6, \gamma, \beta_6) \tag{6.6}$$

in which $z \in Z = [0, 100]$, while $\alpha_k$, $\beta_k$, $\gamma$ are borders for the fuzzy supports and they also constitute some numbers from the interval [0, 100].

Let us further decide the values of the boundary parameters $\alpha_k$, $\beta_k$, $\gamma$ in order to construct constrains for the fuzzy sets that represent the terms of the mentioned list "the curative drug effectiveness regarding a symptom".

### Example 6.1

We suggest the following linear functions that can be approved as the membership functions of terms constituting the contents of the effectiveness list

$$\mu_{R_1}(z) = \mu_{\text{"none"}}(z) = 1 - L(z, 0, 20),$$
$$\mu_{R_2}(z) = \mu_{\text{"almost none"}}(z) = 1 - L(z, 10, 30),$$
$$\mu_{R_3}(z) = \mu_{\text{"very little"}}(z) = 1 - L(z, 20, 40),$$
$$\mu_{R_4}(z) = \mu_{\text{"little"}}(z) = 1 - L(z, 30, 50),$$
$$\mu_{R_5}(z) = \mu_{\text{"rather little"}}(z) = 1 - L(z, 40, 60),$$
$$\mu_{R_6}(z) = \mu_{\text{"medium"}}(z) = \pi(z, 30, 50, 70),$$
$$\mu_{R_7}(z) = \mu_{\text{"rather large"}}(z) = L(z, 40, 60),$$
$$\mu_{R_8}(z) = \mu_{\text{"large"}}(z) = L(z, 50, 70),$$
$$\mu_{R_9}(z) = \mu_{\text{"very large"}}(z) = L(z, 60, 80),$$
$$\mu_{R_{10}}(z) = \mu_{\text{"almost complete"}}(z) = L(z, 70, 90),$$
$$\mu_{R_{11}}(z) = \mu_{\text{"complete"}}(z) = L(z, 80, 100)$$

for $z \in [0, 100]$.

The parameters $\alpha_k$, $\beta_k$ and $\gamma$ in equations above have been proposed in conformity with the physician's suggestion. In order to give an image of the restrictions' appearance we sketch them in Fig. 6.1.

The membership functions presented in Ex. 6.1 can be adopted as a foundation of other fuzzy sets, this time finite sets corresponding to $R_1$–$R_{11}$. To accomplish a process of generating a class of discrete sets, replacing $R_1$–$R_{11}$, we take only the essential parts of sets into consideration, i.e., the elements of their supports that possess membership degrees greater than 0.5. The continuous membership functions serve as a tool for calculating the membership degrees of some of the chosen elements coming from the set supports.

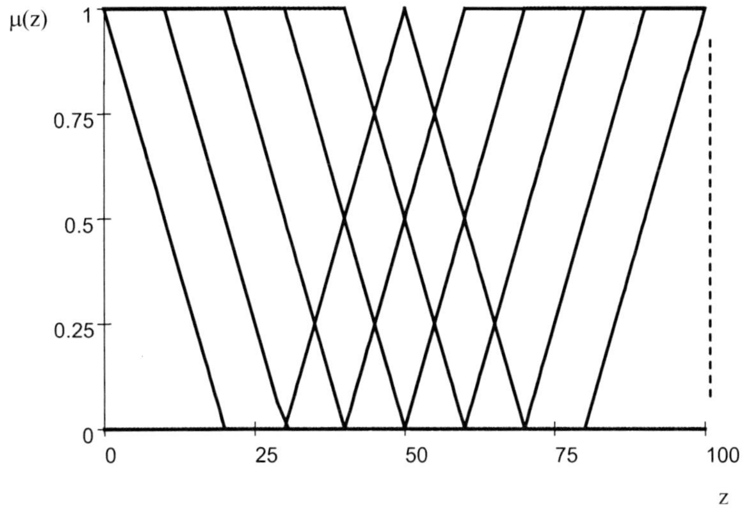


Figure 6.1: The fuzzy constraints $R_1$–$R_{11}$

**Example 6.2**

By involving the patterns from Ex. 6.1, we form the following discrete fuzzy sets, which act on behalf of $R_1$–$R_{11}$

$$R_1 = \text{"}none\text{"} = 1/0 + 0.9/2 + 0.8/4 + 0.7/6 + 0.6/8,$$

$$R_2 = \text{"}almost\ none\text{"} = 1/10 + 0.9/12 + 0.8/14 + 0.7/16 + 0.6/18,$$

$$R_3 = \text{"}very\ little\text{"} = 1/20 + 0.9/22 + 0.8/24 + 0.7/26 + 0.6/28,$$

$$R_4 = \text{"}little\text{"} = 1/30 + 0.9/32 + 0.8/34 + 0.7/36 + 0.6/38,$$

$$R_5 = \text{"}rather\ little\text{"} = 1/40 + 0.9/42 + 0.8/44 + 0.7/46 + 0.6/48,$$

$$R_6 = \text{"}medium\text{"} = 0.6/42 + 0.7/44 + 0.8/46 + 0.9/48 + 1/50 + 0.9/52 + 0.8/54 + 0.7/56 + 0.6/58,$$

$$R_7 = \text{"}rather\ large\text{"} = 0.6/52 + 0.7/54 + 0.8/56 + 0.9/58 + 1/60,$$

$$R_8 = \text{"}large\text{"} = 0.6/62 + 0.7/64 + 0.8/66 + 0.9/68 + 1/70,$$

$$R_9 = \text{"}very\ large = 0.6/72 + 0.7/74 + 0.8/76 + 0.9/78 + 1/80,$$

$$R_{10} = \text{"}almost\ complete\text{"} = {}^{0.6}\!/_{82} + {}^{0.7}\!/_{84} + {}^{0.8}\!/_{86} + {}^{0.9}\!/_{88} + {}^{1}\!/_{90},$$

$$R_{11} = \text{"}complete\text{"} = {}^{0.6}\!/_{92} + {}^{0.7}\!/_{94} + {}^{0.8}\!/_{96} + {}^{0.9}\!/_{98} + {}^{1}\!/_{100}.$$

The fuzzy sets $U_{ij}$ from the utility matrix $U$ can be now replaced by the built fuzzy sets $R_1$–$R_{11}$. To state a connection between $a_i$ (medicine) and the effectiveness of the retreat of $x_j$ (symptom) the physician uses the word from the list "the curative drug effectiveness regarding a symptom" and this word is "translated" into the fuzzy set $R_k$, $k = 1, 2, \ldots, 11$.

Let us also admit that the physician possesses a general experience as to the "difficulties" in the remission of the symptoms $x_j$, $j = 1, 2, \ldots, m$. His medical knowledge, based on observations, can contribute in a classification of symptoms that are harder to treat, and those symptoms that recede more readily during the treatment process. Via the words from the list, "the curative drug effectiveness regarding a symptom", one may assign to each symptom a general ability to retreat, fixed, for instance, by observing the cure of many patients with different drugs. For instance, it is commonly known that a fever disappears quicker than some changes in tissues after inflammation. Such an average classification of symptoms found its place in the fuzzy set $S$ defined theoretically by (6.2), in which the membership degrees $\mu_S(x_j)$, $j = 1, 2, \ldots, m$, correspond now to the fuzzy sets $R_k$, $k = 1, 2, \ldots, 11$. These express the mean effectiveness of treatment independently of a prescribed medicine. By the "cure", one can mean the level of the retreating symptom, the decrease of the heightened index, and the like.

In accordance with Jain's theory of decision-making, the fuzzy utility [38, 39, 40, 59, 60, 62] for each decision-drug $a_i$, $i = 1, 2, \ldots, n$, with the fuzzy state $S \subseteq X$ characterized by means of the membership degrees $\mu_S(x_j)$ is defined to be the set

$$U_i = {}^{\mu_S(x_1)}\!/_{U_{i1}} + {}^{\mu_S(x_2)}\!/_{U_{i2}} + \cdots + {}^{\mu_S(x_m)}\!/_{U_{im}} \tag{6.7}$$

for $i = 1, 2, \ldots, n$. The set allows observing the relationship between the general ability to soothe, and this effect in soothing which the drug $a_i$ causes for each symptom $x_j$. Both the membership degrees $\mu_S(x_j)$ and the elements $U_{ij}$ in the support of the set $U_i$ are the fuzzy sets of the discrete type $R_1$–$R_{11}$.

It is not possible to make further calculations on such sets that have fuzzy sets as the elements of supports and the membership degrees. We thus need an operation that reduces this family of fuzzy sets to one fuzzy set. This is grounded on the single support with clearly determined membership degrees. We test a concatenation operator [59, 62]

$$U_i = \sum_{j=1}^{m} \mu_S(x_j) \Big/ U_{ij} = \sum_{x_j \in X} \sum_{t=1}^{r} \mu_{R_{k\phi}}(z_t) \Big/ z_t \Bigg/ \sum_{c=1}^{q} \mu_{R_{k\varphi}}(z_c) \Big/ z_c =$$

$$= \sum_{\substack{(z_t, z_c) \in \\ \{z_1, z_2, \ldots, z_r\} \\ \times \\ \{z_1, z_2, \ldots, z_q\}}} \min(\mu_{R_{k\phi}}(z_t), \mu_{R_{k\varphi}}(z_c)) \Bigg/ \frac{z_t + z_c}{2} = \sum_{z \in Z} \mu_{U_i}(z) \Big/ z \tag{6.8}$$

in which $\mu_S(x_j)$ is the equal of a fuzzy set $\sum_{t=1}^{r} \mu_{R_{k\phi}}(z_t) \Big/ z_t$ while $U_{ij}$ is another fuzzy set given as $\sum_{c=1}^{q} \mu_{R_{k\varphi}}(z_c) \Big/ z_c$ for $R_{k_\phi}$ and $R_{k_\varphi}$ belonging to the class of the sets $R_1$–$R_{11}$. Each $U_{ij}$ expresses the fuzzy utility following the decision $a_i$ with the result $x_j$. However, by $\mu_S(x_j)$ we judge if $x_j$ is a symptom having a tendency to disappear.

When the same element $z$ in the support of the fuzzy set appears with different membership degrees $\mu_1(z)$ and $\mu_2(z)$, we will aggregate their values by adopting the Jain operation

$$\mu_1(z) \oplus \mu_2(z) = \mu_1(z) + \mu_2(z) - \mu_1(z) \cdot \mu_2(z) . \tag{6.9}$$

The sign "⊕" denotes a symbolic addition of two different membership degrees assigned to the same support element.

**Example 6.3**

Suppose that $A = 0.8/2 + 0.4/3 + 0.5/2 + 0.2/2 + 1/3$. Since the support members $x$ = 2, 3 appear more than once then we should rearrange $A$ due to the following operations

$$A = 0.8/2 + 0.4/3 + 0.5/2 + 0.2/2 + 1/3 = 0.8 + 0.5 - 0.8 \cdot 0.5/2 + 0.2/2$$
$$+ 0.4 + 1 - 0.4 \cdot 1/3 = 0.9/2 + 0.2/2 + 1/3 = 0.9 + 0.2 - 0.9 \cdot 0.2/2 + 1/3$$
$$= 0.92/2 + 1/3 .$$

We notice that this sort of a concatenation operation, recommended by (6.9), raises the aggregated values of membership degrees computed for the same elements in the support of a fuzzy set when comparing them to primary values. We will employ the operations of the (6.9) type to induce the most optimistic prognosis in further investigations.

### 6.2.2 The Solution of Jain's Decision Case

The problem of choosing an optimal decision is solved according to the algorithm developed by Jain [38, 39]. The steps of the action line are listed in the following order.

**Algorithm 6.1**

1. We form a non-fuzzy set $Y$ as the union of supports characteristic of $U_i$, $i = 1, 2, \ldots, n$. This set contains the elements $z \in Z$, which appear in all sets $U_i$. Hence, we have access to the range of the common utility expressed as $Y = \bigcup_{i=1}^{n} \text{supp}(U_i)$.
2. We select the maximal element of the set $Y$, so-called $z_{\max}$.
3. We define the fuzzy sets $U_i'$ as

$$U_i' = \sum_{z \in Z} \mu_{U_i'}(z) \Big/ z \tag{6.10}$$

for $z \in \text{supp}(U_i)$. This means that the supports of $U_i'$ and $U_i$ are the same sets. The membership degrees of $U_i'$ are computed by means of the formula

$$\mu_{U_i'}(z) = \frac{z_{U_i}}{z_{\max}}, \tag{6.11}$$

where $z_{U_i}$ stands for an element belonging to the support of the set $U_i$. $U_i'$'s membership degrees evaluate the "deviation" between the elements of $U_i$, and the maximal $z$ found in the union of all $U_i$.
4. The next introduced fuzzy set has the form of

$$U_{i0} = \sum_{z \in Z} \mu_{U_{i0}}(z) \Big/ z, \tag{6.12}$$

provided that the membership degree $\mu_{U_{i0}}(z)$ is calculated according to the rule

$$\mu_{U_{i0}}(z) = \min(\mu_{U_i}(z), \mu_{U_i'}(z)) . \tag{6.13}$$

The fuzzy utility $U_{i0}$, constructed for each medicine $a_i$ gathers all possible factors that can affect appreciation of the soothing power of $a_i$. The minimum operation is used in (6.13) in order to reduce too large values of final results, which as we remember, are effects of the operation ⊕ induced by (6.9).

5. We slowly close the action of Algorithm 6.1 by the adoption of a new fuzzy set $A^*$ composed of elements $a_1, a_2, \ldots, a_n$ ($a_i \in A$, $i = 1, 2, \ldots, n$) and formalized by

$$A^* = \sum_{i=1}^{n} \mu_{A^*}(a_i) \Big/ a_i . \tag{6.14}$$

The membership degree for each $a_i$ is generated by

$$\mu_{A^*}(a_i) = \underset{z \in \mathrm{supp}(U_{i0})}{\text{mean value}}(\mu_{U_{i0}}(z)) . \tag{6.15}$$

In practice we compute the arithmetic mean for a sample of membership degrees appearing in each set $U_{i0}$. This value expresses the decisive character of every $a_i$ in accordance with a rule: the higher the value of the membership degree assigned to $a_i$ is, the better the influence of $a_i$ on the patient's health is to be expected.

6. To terminate the choice of an optimal decision $a^*$ we accept as $a^*$ this $a_i$ whose membership degree satisfies the equation

$$\mu_{A^*}(a^*) = \max_{1 \le i \le n}(\mu_{A^*}(a_i)) , \tag{6.16}$$

and we ascertain that the application of the drug $a^*$ should yield the best effects in the retreating process of the symptoms $x_j$, $j = 1, 2, \ldots, m$.

**Example 6.4**

The Jain model is tested on the clinical data coming from the investigation carried out among patients who suffer from $D$ = "*coronary heart disease*". We consider the most typical symptoms accompanying the illness, i.e., $x_1$ = "*pain in chest*", $x_2$ = "*changes in ECG*", and $x_3$ = "*increased level of LDL-cholesterol*". A physician has recommended $a_1$ = *nitroglycerin*, $a_2$ = *beta-adrenergic blockade*, $a_3$ = *acetylsalicylic acid* (*aspirin*) and $a_4$ = *statine LDL-reductor* as the medicines expected to improve the patient's state. The physician has also decided that the set $S$ and the matrix $U$ should have the following descriptions

$$S = {}^{large}\!/_{x_1} + {}^{medium}\!/_{x_2} + {}^{rather\ large}\!/_{x_3}$$

and

$$U = \begin{array}{c} \\ a_1 \\ a_2 \\ a_3 \\ a_4 \end{array} \begin{array}{c} \begin{array}{ccc} x_1 & x_2 & x_3 \end{array} \\ \begin{bmatrix} complete & very\ large & almost\ none \\ medium & medium & little \\ little & little & very\ little \\ little & little & very\ large \end{bmatrix} \end{array}.$$

We begin the computations with determining supports of the sets $U_i$. For instance, the set $U_1$ is decided as

$$U_1 = {}^{large}\!/_{complete} + {}^{medium}\!/_{very\ large} + {}^{rather\ large}\!/_{almost\ none} =$$

$$\frac{0.6/62 + \cdots + 1/70}{0.6/92 + \cdots + 1/100} + \frac{0.6/42 + \cdots + 1/50 + \cdots + 0.6/58}{0.6/72 + \cdots + 1/80} +$$

$$\frac{0.6/52 + \cdots + 1/60}{1/10 + \cdots + 0.6/18} =$$

$$\min(0.6,0.6)\Big/\tfrac{62+92}{2} + \cdots + \min(1,1)\Big/\tfrac{70+100}{2} + \min(0.6,0.6)\Big/\tfrac{42+72}{2} + \cdots + \min(0.6,1)\Big/\tfrac{58+80}{2} +$$

$$\min(0.6,1)\Big/\tfrac{52+10}{2} + \cdots + \min(1,0.6)\Big/\tfrac{60+18}{2} =$$

$$0.6/31 + 0.88/32 + 0.938/33 + 0.998/34 + 0.964/35 + 0.998/36 + 0.976/37 + 0.88/38 +$$

$$0.6/39 + 0.6/57 + 0.84/58 + 0.952/59 + 0.986/60 + 0.997/61 + 0.9986/62 + 0.997/63 +$$

$$0.999/64 + 0.1/65 + 0.998/66 + 0.9761/67 + 0.88/68 + 0.6/69 + 0.6/77 + 0.84/78 +$$

$$0.952/79 + 0.974/80 + 0.998/81 + 0.999/82 + 0.988/83 + 0.999/84 + 1/85$$

when applying (6.8) and (6.9).

By repeating the procedure developed above we obtain the sets

$$U_2 = 0.6/41 + 0.952/42 + 0.976/43 + 0.998/44 + 1/45 + 0.998/46 + 0.97/47 + 0.988/48 + 0.6/49 + 1/50 + 0.96/52 + 0.84/53 + 0.99/54 + 0.986/55 + 0.999/56 + 0.998/57 + 0.998/58 + 0.999/59 + 1/60 + 0.992/61 + 0.976/62 + 0.88/63 + 0.6/64,$$

$$U_3 = 0.84/36 + 0.986/37 + 0.999/38 + 0.999/39 + 1/40 + 0.999/41 + 0.999/42 + 0.999/43 + 0.999/44 + 0.986/45 + 0.98/46 + 0.994/47 + 0.99/48 + 0.992/49 + 1/50 + 0.992/51 + 0.976/52 + 0.88/53 + 0.6/54$$

and

$$U_4 = 0.6/36 + 0.88/37 + 0.976/38 + 0.99/39 + 1/40 + 0.999/41 + 0.999/42 + 0.998/43 + 0.998/44 + 0.986/45 + 0.98/46 + 0.98/47 + 0.984/48 + 0.992/49 + 1/50 + 0.992/51 + 0.976/52 + 0.88/53 + 0.6/54 + 0.6/62 + 0.84/63 + 0.952/64 + 0.986/65 + 0.998/66 + 0.998/67 + 0.976/68 + 0.99/69 + 1/70\,.$$

The non-fuzzy sum of all supports emerges as a set

$$\bigcup_{i=1}^{4} \mathrm{supp}(U_i) =$$

{31, 32, 33, 34, 35, 36, 37, 38, 39, 40, 41, 42, 43, 44, 45, 46, 47, 48, 49, 50, 51, 52, 53, 54, 55, 56, 57, 58, 59, 60, 61, 62, 63, 64, 65, 66, 67, 68, 69, 70, 77, 78, 79, 80, 81, 82, 83, 84, 85}

in which the largest element is found as $z_{\max} = 85$.

Equations (6.10) and (6.11) give rise to the creation of new sets $U_i'$, $i$ = 1, 2, 3, 4. $U_1'$ – the first set in the sequence – appears as the following fuzzy collection of elements

$$U_1' = \frac{31}{85}\Big/31 + \frac{32}{85}\Big/32 + \frac{33}{85}\Big/33 + \cdots + \frac{84}{85}\Big/84 + \frac{85}{85}\Big/85 =$$
$$0.36/31 + 0.376/32 + 0.388/33 + 0.4/34 + 0.41/35 + 0.42/36 + 0.435/37 + 0.447/38 +$$
$$0.459/39 + 0.67/57 + 0.682/58 + 0.694/59 + 0.706/60 + 0.718/61 + 0.729/62 +$$
$$0.741/63 + 0.753/64 + 0.765/65 + 0.776/66 + 0.788/67 + 0.8/68 + 0.811/69 +$$
$$0.9/77 + 0.917/78 + 0.929/79 + 0.94/80 + 0.953/82 + 0.965/82 + 0.976/83 +$$
$$0.988/84 + 1/85 .$$

The other sets of $U_1'$'s type, $i = 2, 3, 4$, are expanded as

$$U_2' = 0.48/41 + 0.494/42 + 0.506/43 + 0.517/44 + 0.529/45 + 0.54/46 + 0.553/47 +$$
$$0.565/48 + 0.576/49 + 0.588/50 + 0.612/52 + 0.623/53 + 0.635/54 + 0.647/55 +$$
$$0.659/56 + 0.67/57 + 0.682/58 + 0.694/59 + 0.706/60 + 0.718/61 + 0.729/62 +$$
$$0.741/63 + 0.753/64 ,$$

$$U_3' = 0.42/36 + 0.435/37 + 0.447/38 + 0.459/39 + 0.470/40 + 0.482/41 + 0.494/42 +$$
$$0.506/43 + 0.518/44 + 0.529/45 + 0.541/46 + 0.553/47 + 0.564/48 + 0.576/49 +$$
$$0.588/50 + 0.6/51 + 0.612/52 + 0.623/53 + 0.635/54$$

and

$$U_4' = 0.42/36 + 0.435/37 + 0.447/38 + 0.459/39 + 0.470/40 + 0.482/41 + 0.494/42 +$$
$$0.506/43 + 0.518/44 + 0.529/45 + 0.541/46 + 0.553/47 + 0.564/48 + 0.576/49 +$$
$$0.588/50 + 0.6/51 + 0.612/52 + 0.623/53 + 0.635/54 + 0.729/62 + 0.741/63 +$$
$$0.753/64 + 0.765/65 + 0.776/66 + 0.788/67 + 0.8/68 + 0.811/69 + 0.823/70 .$$

We follow the next step of Algorithm 6.1 to arrange the sets $U_{i0}$, $i = 1, 2, 3, 4$ as

$$U_{10} = \frac{\min(0.6,0.36)}{31} + \frac{\min(0.88,0.376)}{32} + \cdots + \frac{\min(1,1)}{85} = 0.36/31 + 0.376/32 + 0.388/33 + 0.4/34 + 0.41/35 + 0.42/36 + 0.435/37 + 0.447/38 + 0.459/39 + 0.6/57 + 0.682/58 + 0.694/59 + 0.706/60 + 0.718/61 + 0.729/62 + 0.741/63 + 0.753/64 + 0.765/65 + 0.776/66 + 0.788/67 + 0.8/68 + 0.6/69 + 0.6/77 + 0.84/78 + 0.929/79 + 0.94/80 + 0.953/81 + 0.965/82 + 0.976/83 + 0.988/84 + 1/85,$$

$$U_{20} = 0.48/41 + 0.494/42 + 0.506/43 + 0.517/44 + 0.529/45 + 0.541/46 + 0.553/47 + 0.565/48 + 0.576/49 + 0.588/50 + 0.612/52 + 0.623/53 + 0.635/54 + 0.647/55 + 0.659/56 + 0.67/57 + 0.682/58 + 0.694/59 + 0.706/60 + 0.718/61 + 0.729/62 + 0.741/63 + 0.6/64,$$

$$U_{30} = 0.42/36 + 0.435/37 + 0.447/38 + 0.459/39 + 0.470/40 + 0.482/41 + 0.494/42 + 0.506/43 + 0.518/44 + 0.529/45 + 0.541/46 + 0.553/47 + 0.564/48 + 0.576/49 + 0.588/50 + 0.6/51 + 0.612/52 + 0.623/53 + 0.6/54$$

and

$$U_{40} = 0.42/36 + 0.435/37 + 0.447/38 + 0.459/39 + 0.470/40 + 0.482/41 + 0.494/42 + 0.506/43 + 0.518/44 + 0.529/45 + 0.541/46 + 0.553/47 + 0.564/48 + 0.576/49 + 0.588/50 + 0.6/51 + 0.612/52 + 0.623/53 + 0.6/54 + 0.6/62 + 0.741/63 + 0.753/64 + 0.765/65 + 0.776/66 + 0.788/67 + 0.8/68 + 0.811/69 + 0.823/70.$$

The decision set $A^*$ has been decided as

$$A^* = \frac{\text{mean}(0.36,0,376,\ldots,1)}{a_1} + \frac{\text{mean}(0.48,0.494,\ldots,0.6)}{a_2} + \frac{\text{mean}(0.42,0.435,\ldots,0.6)}{a_3} + \frac{\text{mean}(0.42,0.435,\ldots,0.823)}{a_4} = 0.685/a_1 + 0.611/a_2 + 0.527/a_3 + 0.603/a_4.$$

The magnitudes of the membership degrees give us a hint about priorities of drugs, i.e., $a_1$ should have the strongest soothing power when regarding the considered symptoms, and it should be accepted as the optimal decision-drug. Moreover, we can state the hierarchy of drugs in the following order: $a_1 \succ a_2 \succ a_4 \succ a_3$. The notion $a_i \succ a_j$ indicates that $a_i$ acts better than $a_j$, $i, j = 1, 2, 3, 4$.

## 6.3 Group Decision-Making in the Selection of Drugs

We have followed the procedure of comparing the healing effect of medicines on the condition that some descriptions, which concern the decisive character of the pairs "*drug – symptom*", are made by one physician. Nevertheless, everyone knows that such opinions are often shared. If we involve several physicians in a discussion about the drug priority, then we can experience that they will hold different views about the curative power of considered medicines. In this section we will give a piece of information about a new technique contributing in the choice of an optimal medicine in spite of contradictory judgements.

Each physician treated as a decision-maker would like to create the matrix $U$ and the set $S$ according to his own experience and judgement. As a result, we obtain different priorities in the set $A^*$. How shall we choose the best medicine in the case when the sets $A^*$ differ a greatly from each other? The question is answered by means of the algorithm based on graphs [40]. We thus adapt the theoretical graph model to a medical task that is sketched below [62].

Let us state a set of physicians $P = \{P_1, P_2, ..., P_t\}$ who appreciate the drugs belonging to set $A = \{a_1, a_2, ..., a_n\}$. A fuzzy relation $\Re \subset A \times A$ with the membership function $\mu_\Re : A \times A \to [0,1]$, called the group order, is represented by membership degrees $\mu_\Re(a_i, a_j)$. These, in turn, appreciate the intensity grade of preference concerning decision $a_i$ in comparison with $a_j$. If we define

$$\delta_{ij} = \{P_s : P_s \quad tells \quad that \quad a_i \succ a_j\}, \tag{6.17}$$

$s = 1, 2, \ldots, t$, $i, j = 1, 2, \ldots, n$, then we will generate membership degrees in relation $\Re$ as

$$\mu_\Re(a_i, a_j) = \frac{|\delta_{ij}|}{t}. \tag{6.18}$$

We now need a definition for the $\alpha$-level of a fuzzy set and apply it in the further part of the discussed many-decision-making-model [12, 40, 95].

**Definition 6.1**

For a fuzzy set $A = \{(x, \mu_A(x))\}$, $x \in X$, we determine a non-fuzzy set

$$A_\alpha = \{x : \mu_A(x) \geq \alpha\}, \quad (6.19)$$

called the $\alpha$-level of $A$.

**Example 6.5**

Suppose that $A = {}^{0.1}\!/_1 + {}^{0.2}\!/_2 + {}^{0.4}\!/_3 + {}^{0.5}\!/_4 + {}^{0.7}\!/_5 + {}^{0.8}\!/_7 + {}^{0.9}\!/_8 + {}^{1}\!/_9 + {}^{0.6}\!/_{10}$ in $X = \{1, \ldots, 10\}$. If $\alpha = 0.4$ then $A_{0.4} = \{3, 4, 5, 7, 8, 9, 10\}$.

For $A$ given by the membership function $\mu_A(x) = \pi(x, 20, 50)$ we state, e.g., $A_{0.5} = [40, 60]$ in accordance with Fig. 6.2.

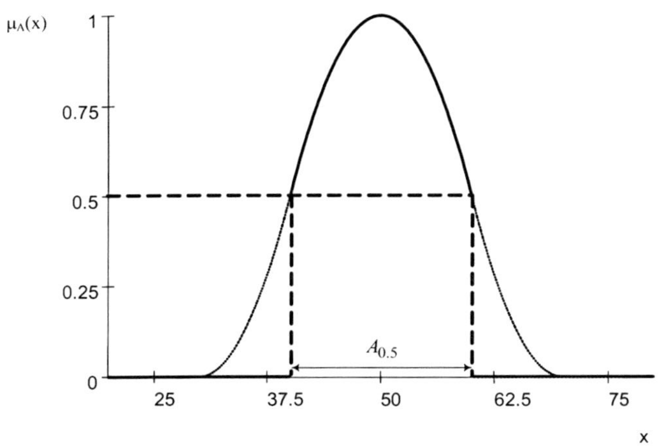


Figure 6.2: The 0.5-level of $A$ characterized by $\pi(x, 20, 50)$

Analogously, the $\alpha$-level $R_\alpha$ of the relation $\Re$ is decided as the set

$$R_\alpha = \{(a_i, a_j) : \mu_\Re(a_i, a_j) \geq \alpha\}. \quad (6.20)$$

For the greatest $\alpha$ we seek a set $R_\alpha$ that contains all decisions $a_i$ and is totally ordered. We treat $a_i$ values as vertices in a directed graph. The order in the pair ($a_i$, $a_j$) indicates the direction of the arrow that ties $a_i$ and $a_j$ together. We should explain that the order in the graph is interpreted as total if each pair of nodes has a connection formed by the arrow. The vertex, that concentrates the most endpoints of the arrows in accordance with $R_\alpha$, is determined as a group decision.

The steps that follow the determination procedure of selecting an optimal medicine are collected in the algorithm developed below.

**Algorithm 6.2**

1. Find "α values"= $\{\mu_{\Re}(a_i,a_j):\mu_{\Re}(a_i,a_j)$ are different in $\Re\} = \{\alpha_1,\alpha_2, ..., \alpha_p\}$ as a set of values arranged in the descending order.
2. Set $k = 1$.
3. Find $R_{\alpha_k}$, $k = 1, \ldots, p$, and sketch a directed graph for $R_{\alpha_k}$ due to the pair order. The notation $a_i \succ a_j$ corresponds to the ordered pair ($a_i$, $a_j$) generating the direction $a_i \leftarrow a_j$.
4. Is the order in $R_{\alpha_k}$ total? →No. Set $k=k+1$. Go To Step 3
   →Yes. Choose the vertex with the largest number of arrow endpoints as an optimal decision

**Example 6.6**

In order to test the group decision model of choosing the best medicine among the four drugs already introduced by Ex. 6.4, we have asked six physicians $P_1$, $P_2$, …, $P_6$ for evaluating the curative effects of the drugs: $a_1$, $a_2$, $a_3$, $a_4$. The medicines, as we remember, show a healing power in "*coronary heart disease*". The priority levels are listed in the following schedule:

$$P_1 = P_3 = P_4 = (a_1 \succ a_2 \succ a_4 \succ a_3),$$
$$P_2 = (a_1 \succ a_4 \succ a_2 \succ a_3),$$
$$P_5 = (a_2 \succ a_1 \succ a_4 \succ a_3),$$
$$P_6 = (a_2 \succ a_4 \succ a_1 \succ a_3).$$

We adopt (6.18) to decide the contents of the matrix $\Re$ as

$$\Re = \begin{array}{c} \\ a_1 \\ a_2 \\ a_3 \\ a_4 \end{array} \begin{array}{c} \begin{array}{cccc} a_1 & a_2 & a_3 & a_4 \end{array} \\ \begin{bmatrix} 0 & 0.67 & 1 & 0.83 \\ 0.33 & 0 & 1 & 0.83 \\ 0 & 0 & 0 & 0 \\ 0.17 & 0.17 & 1 & 0 \end{bmatrix} \end{array}.$$

The "α-values" set is sorted as "α-values" = {1, 0.83, 0.67, 0.33, 0.17}.

For $k = 1$ we find $R_1 = \{(a_1,a_3),(a_2,a_3),(a_4,a_3)\}$. The associated graph $R_1$, plotted in Fig. 6.3, does not reveal the total order.

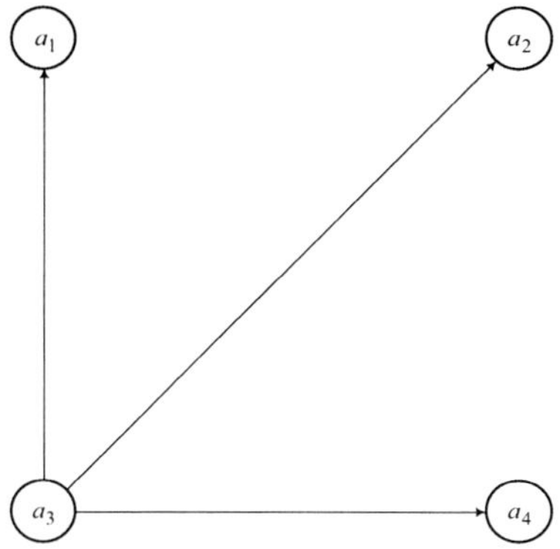


Figure 6.3: The set $R_1$ as the directed graph

If $k = 2$ we set $R_{0.83} = \{(a_1,a_3),(a_2,a_3),(a_4,a_3),(a_1,a_4),(a_2,a_4)\}$ that constitutes a basis of the graph $R_{0.83}$ presented in Fig. 6.4.

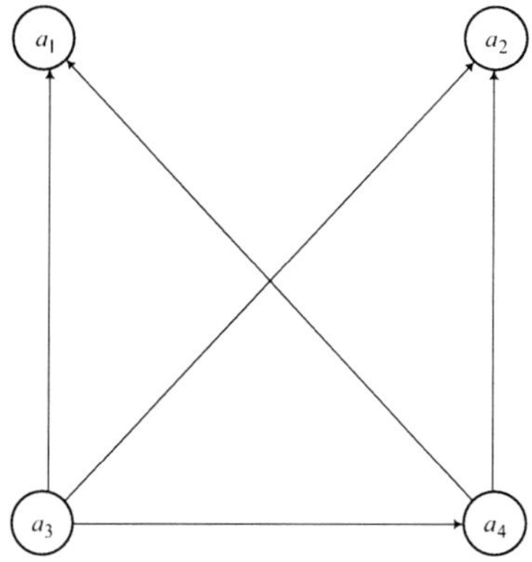


Figure 6.4: The set $R_{0.83}$ as the directed graph

The graph $R_{0.83}$ has not the total order either, since the pair ($a_1$, $a_2$) is lacking a connection.

We thus prove if the set $R_{0.67} = \{(a_1,a_3),(a_2,a_3),(a_4,a_3),(a_1,a_4),(a_2,a_4),$ $(a_1,a_2)\}$, generating the graph $R_{0.67}$ drawn in Fig. 6.5, will be totally ordered.

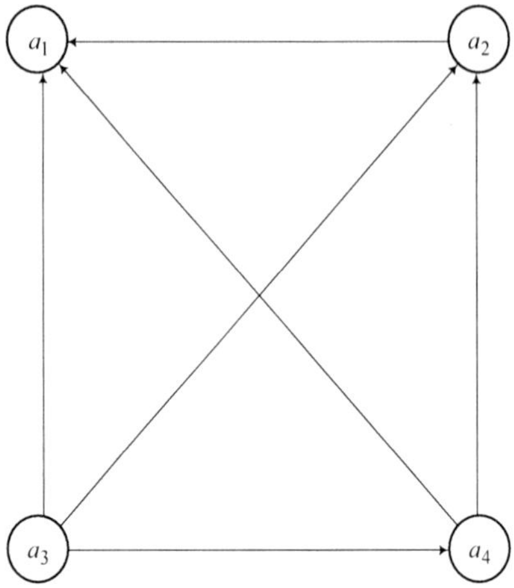


Figure 6.5: The set $R_{0.67}$ as the directed graph

Finally, we have determined the set of pairs that form the total order in the associated graph. By counting the number of arrow endpoints, tended towards each vertex, we should state the group decision concerning a hierarchy of drugs as $a_1 \succ a_2 \succ a_4 \succ a_3$.

The models discussed in Sections 6.2 and 6.3 should be simple for an eventual user since they do not require deep knowledge in making calculations.

In the last models the physicians' data reports have been tested very thoroughly because of introducing the finite fuzzy sets of effectiveness. We want to emphasize that even one value representing the effectiveness – we have numerically stated presence in the diagnostic model in such a way – should yield satisfactory results. However, the occurrence of expressing the effectiveness terms as fuzzy sets, eliminates a risk of casual results and should be admitted by users as a safe decision step. The decisions obtained lately seem to be very reliable in spite of different interactions between the drugs and their influence on the symptoms. The hierarchy of drugs is even debatable when involving many decision-makers in the process of their evaluation. Physicians often share different opinions concerning medicine priorities, but it is still mathematically possible to sum up all conclusions as a final selection of the most efficacious remedy. The obtained results have also been confirmed by experienced pharmacologists.

## 6.4 Unequal Objectives in the Choice of Medicines

The purpose of this section is to present some ideas on the applications of fuzzy sets to multi-objective decision making, with particular emphasis on a means of including differing degrees of importance to different objectives. Different approaches to aggregation of weighted decision criteria have constituted a subject of lively discussions during last decades [5, 13, 21, 57, 80, 83, 85].

The primary reasons for the usefulness of fuzzy sets in handling multi-objectives are: ability to represent objectives, convenient forms for combining objectives and means of including differing degrees of importance to the objectives [81].

### 6.4.1 The Design of Objectives-Constraints

We still consider a decision model in which $n$ drugs $a_1, ..., a_n \in A$ act as decisions. These affect $m$ symptoms $x_1, ..., x_m \in X$ that are typical of a morbid unit under consideration. The drugs-decisions constitute $n$ elements in supports of fuzzy sets $K_t$, $t$ = 1, …, $m$, $m$+1, $m$+2, determined as some criteria-objectives restricting the set $A$. Thus, we can recognize each set $K_t$ as a fuzzy subset of $A$, i.e., $\mu_{K_t} : A \rightarrow [0,1]$, $t = 1, ..., m+2$. In the model of accepting the most optimal medicine $A_i$, $i$ = 1, …, $n$, we assume that some of restriction sets $K_j$, $j$ = 1, …, $m$, are defined by

$$K_j = \text{"influence of } a_1, ..., a_n \text{ on symptom } x_j\text{"} =$$
$$a_1\text{'s } \textit{effectiveness} \text{ regarding } x_j \Big/ a_1 + \cdots + a_n\text{'s } \textit{effectiveness} \text{ regarding } x_j \Big/ a_n \quad . \tag{6.21}$$

In spite of drug effectiveness, which definitely is the most important factor in the appreciation of drug action, we can introduce other important factors assisting drug decision-making like side effects of medicines or their prices. We thus form the following fuzzy sets

$$K_{m+1} = \text{"estimation of } \textit{side effects} \text{ of } a_1, ..., a_n \text{ supporting the decision positively"} =$$
$$1 - \textit{side effects} \text{ of } a_1 \Big/ a_1 + \cdots + 1 - \textit{side effects} \text{ of } a_n \Big/ a_n \tag{6.22}$$

and

$$K_{m+2} = \text{"estimation of } \textit{price availability} \text{ for } a_1, ..., a_n\text{"} =$$
$$\textit{price availability} \text{ of } a_1 \Big/ a_1 + \cdots + \textit{price availability} \text{ of } a_n \Big/ a_n \tag{6.23}$$

in order to enlarge a number of decisive indications.

**Example 6.7**

We return to the clinical data from Ex. 6.4, which concerns $D$ = "*coronary heart disease*". We still consider the symptoms $x_1$ = "*pain in chest*", $x_2$ = "*changes in ECG*" and $x_3$ = "*increased level of LDL-cholesterol*". Even the medicines are unchanged and we list them as $a_1$ = *nitroglycerin*, $a_2$ = *beta-adrenergic blockade*, $a_3$ = *acetylsalicylic acid* (*aspirin*) and $a_4$ = *statine LDL-reductor*.

The procedure of stating effectiveness has been based on fuzzy sets in Ex. 6.2. Nevertheless, even if the mathematical presentation of each effectiveness as a distinct fuzzy set has been very efficient and thorough, we probably do not need such accuracy in determining the sets $K_j$, $j = 1, \ldots, m$, because of concentration on their importance instead. We assign only one value to every effectiveness term that is an approved procedure as shown in Chapter 3. To decide adequate representatives $z \in [0, 100]$ of the effectiveness descriptions from Ex. 6.2, we take, when we return to (6.5), $z = \alpha_k$ for $k = 1, 2, 3, 4, 5$, and $z = \beta_k$ for $k = 7, 8, 9, 10, 11$, respectively $z = \gamma$ for $k = 6$ due to (6.6). On the basis of Ex. 6.1, we select $z$-values, which stand for the exponents of the following expressions: $z_{\text{"none"}} = 0$, $z_{\text{"almost none"}} = 10$, $z_{\text{"very little"}} = 20$, $z_{\text{"little"}} = 30$, $z_{\text{"rather little"}} = 40$, $z_{\text{"medium"}} = 50$, $z_{\text{"rather large"}} = 60$, $z_{\text{"large"}} = 70$, $z_{\text{"very large"}} = 80$, $z_{\text{"almost complete"}} = 90$, $z_{\text{"complete"}} = 100$. If we fit a membership function $\mu_{\text{"effectiveness"}}(z) = L(z,0,100)$ over $[0, 100]$ as recommended by (6.3), we will obtain the final membership values $\mu(z)$ for $z$ sorted above. These replace the terms of effectiveness according to the pattern shown in Table 6.1.

Table 6.1: The representatives of linearly modeled effectiveness terms

| Effectiveness | Representing $z$-value | $\mu(z)$ |
|---|---|---|
| "*none*" | 0 | 0 |
| "*almost none*" | 10 | 0.1 |
| "*very little*" | 20 | 0.2 |
| "*little*" | 30 | 0.3 |
| "*rather little*" | 40 | 0.4 |
| "*medium*" | 50 | 0.5 |
| "*rather large*" | 60 | 0.6 |
| "*large*" | 70 | 0.7 |
| "*very large*" | 80 | 0.8 |
| "*almost complete*" | 90 | 0.9 |
| "*complete*" | 100 | 1 |

We reconstruct the sets $K_j$, $j = 1, 2, 3$, due to (6.21), by applying the columns from the matrix $U$ introduced by Ex. 6.4. Hence

$$K_1 = \text{"influence of } a_1,\ a_2,\ a_3,\ a_4 \text{ on } x_1\text{"} =$$

$$\mathit{complete}/a_1 + \mathit{medium}/a_2 + \mathit{little}/a_3 + \mathit{little}/a_4 =$$

$$1/a_1 + 0.5/a_2 + 0.3/a_3 + 0.3/a_4,$$

$$K_2 = \text{"influence of } a_1, a_2, a_3, a_4 \text{ on } x_2\text{"} =$$
$$\textit{very large}/a_1 + \textit{medium}/a_2 + \textit{little}/a_3 + \textit{little}/a_4 =$$
$$0.8/a_1 + 0.5/a_2 + 0.3/a_3 + 0.3/a_4$$

and

$$K_3 = \text{"influence of } a_1, a_2, a_3, a_4 \text{ on } x_3\text{"} =$$
$$\textit{almost none}/a_1 + \textit{little}/a_2 + \textit{very little}/a_3 + \textit{very large}/a_4 =$$
$$0.1/a_1 + 0.3/a_2 + 0.2/a_3 + 0.8/a_4 .$$

The physician has estimated side effects of the drugs in the set $K_4$ by assimilating the words from the first columns of Table 6.4. The side effects of $a_i$, $i = 1, \ldots, n$, are rather unfavorable occurrences; therefore their lack in $a_i$, e.g., "*side effects* of $a_i$" = "*almost none*", should be emphasized by the larger membership value assigned to $a_i$ as an indication of safe medicine consumption. For the purpose of enlarging membership values of these medicines that do not have side effects, we use the complement operation 1 – estimation of *side effects*. Set $K_4$ is established in accordance with (6.22) as

$$K_4 = \text{"estimation of } \textit{side effects} \text{ of } a_1, a_2, a_3, a_4 \text{ supporting the decision positively"} =$$
$$1 - \textit{very little}/a_1 + 1 - \textit{little}/a_2 + 1 - \textit{rather large}/a_3 + 1 - \textit{very little}/a_4 =$$
$$1-0.2/a_1 + 1-0.3/a_2 + 1-0.6/a_3 + 1-0.2/a_4 = 0.8/a_1 + 0.7/a_2 + 0.4/a_3 + 0.8/a_4 .$$

The prices of all medicines are not in the least inconvenient for patients to purchase them. Thus, if we note that the large value of a membership degree corresponds to a rather cheap and available medicine we can state the set $K_5$ by adopting (6.23) as

$$K_5 = \text{"estimation of } \textit{price availability} \text{ for } a_1, a_2, a_3, a_4\text{"} =$$
$$0.8/a_1 + 0.8/a_2 + 0.9/a_3 + 0.8/a_4 .$$

After preparing the criteria-objectives we are ready to make a fuzzy decision, which is affected by all of them.

The fuzzy decision $D$, which takes into account $K_1$ and $K_2$ and … and $K_{m+2}$ is made in accordance with the minimum decision rule [9, 40]

$$D = K_1 \cap K_2 \cap \cdots \cap K_m \cap \cdots \cap K_{m+2} \,. \tag{6.24}$$

This provides us with the membership function

$$\mu_D(a_i) = \min(\mu_{K_1}(a_i), \mu_{K_2}(a_i), \ldots, \mu_{K_m}(a_i), \ldots, \mu_{K_{m+2}}(a_i)) \tag{6.25}$$

for each $a_i \in A$.

The optimal drug-decision is accepted as this $a_i$, $i = 1, \ldots, n$, which has the maximal value of the membership degree in $D$ as defined by (6.16).

### 6.4.2 The Power-Importance of Objectives

If we can associate with each fuzzy objective $K_t$, $t = 1, \ldots, m, m+1, m+2$, a non negative number that indicates its power or importance in the decision according to the rule: the higher the number the more important criterion $K_t$, then we could raise each fuzzy criterion set to this power before combining to form $D$. We regard $w_1, w_2, \ldots, w_m, \ldots, w_{m+2}$ as powers-weights of $K_1, K_2, \ldots, K_m, \ldots, K_{m+2}$ to modify (6.24) as a richer and more extended decision

$$D = K_1^{w_1} \cap K_2^{w_2} \cap \cdots \cap K_m^{w_m} \cap \cdots \cap K_{m+2}^{w_{m+2}} \tag{6.26}$$

in which the membership degree of each $a_i \in A$ is determined as

$$\mu_D(a_i) = \min((\mu_{K_1}(a_i))^{w_1}, (\mu_{K_2}(a_i))^{w_2}, \ldots, (\mu_{K_m}(a_i))^{w_m}, \ldots, (\mu_{K_{m+2}}(a_i))^{w_{m+2}}). \tag{6.27}$$

We note that each $K_t$ always takes the values of membership degrees from [0, 1]. If $w_t$ gets bigger then $(\mu_{K_t}(a_i))^{w_t}$, $t = 1, \ldots, m, \ldots, m + 2$, $i = 1, \ldots, n$, will get smaller, closer to zero. On the contrary, $w_t \to 0$ implies $(\mu_{K_t}(a_i))^{w_t} \to 1$. This behaviour of $K_t$'s membership degrees emphasizes that the choice of the minimum operation in (6.27) is proper. The membership grade in all objectives having little importance ($w_t < 1$) becomes larger, and while those in objectives having more importance ($w_t > 1$) become smaller. Since we use the minimum operation to the membership degrees in the decision set $D$, we will exclude the larger values that are rather unimportant. This has the effect of making the membership function of the decision set $D$ as useful in the decision making process as possible when taking care of all decisive factors.

A procedure for obtaining a ratio scale of importance for a group of $m + 2$ elements (like in the drug-decision model) was developed by Saaty [68].

Assume that we have $m + 2$ objectives and we want to construct a scale, rating these objectives as to their importance with respect to the decision. We ask a decision-maker to compare the objectives in paired comparison. If we are comparing objective $t$ with objective $l$, we assign the values $b_{tl}$ and $b_{lt}$ as follows

(1) $b_{lt} = \dfrac{1}{b_{tl}}$.

(2) If objective $t$ is more important than objective $l$ then $b_{tl}$ gets assigned a number according to the following scheme:

| *Intensity of importance expressed by the value of* $b_{tl}$ | *Definition* |
|---|---|
| 1 | Equal importance of $K_t$ and $K_l$ |
| 3 | Weak importance of $K_t$ over $K_l$ |
| 5 | Strong importance of $K_t$ over $K_l$ |
| 7 | Demonstrated importance of $K_t$ over $K_l$ |
| 9 | Absolute importance of $K_t$ over $K_l$ |
| 2, 4, 6, 8 | Intermediate values |

If objective $l$ is more important than objective $t$, we assign the value of $b_{lt}$.

Having obtained the above judgments an $(m + 2) \times (m + 2)$ importance matrix $B$ is constructed in the drug decision problem sketched above.

**Example 6.8**

By involving the computation technique suggested in the description of matrix $B$ we try to find the weights for objectives $K_t$, $t = 1, \ldots, 5$, already stated in Ex. 6.7.

The physical status of a patient is subjectively better if the pain disappears that means that a physician tries to release the patient from symptom $x_1$ = "*pain in chest*". The next priority is assigned to $x_2$ = "*changes in ECG*" and finally, we concentrate our attention on getting rid of $x_3$ = "*increased level of LDL-cholesterol*". The last symptom does not disappear very quickly and the patient must be treated for some time to be free from it.

These remarks are helpful when constructing a content of the matrix $B$ as

$$B = \begin{array}{c} \\ K_1 \\ K_2 \\ K_3 \\ K_4 \\ K_5 \end{array} \begin{array}{c} \begin{array}{ccccc} K_1 & K_2 & K_3 & K_4 & K_5 \end{array} \\ \begin{bmatrix} 1 & 3 & 5 & 7 & 7 \\ \frac{1}{3} & 1 & 3 & 7 & 7 \\ \frac{1}{5} & \frac{1}{3} & 1 & 7 & 7 \\ \frac{1}{7} & \frac{1}{7} & \frac{1}{7} & 1 & 3 \\ \frac{1}{7} & \frac{1}{7} & \frac{1}{7} & \frac{1}{3} & 1 \end{bmatrix} \end{array}.$$

Matrix $B$ constitutes a crucial part in the procedure of determining the degrees of importance $w_1, \ldots, w_m, \ldots, w_{m+2}$ that affect the decision set $D$ in a substantial way (in accord with (6.27)). The weights are decided as components of this eigen vector which corresponds to the largest in magnitude eigen value of the matrix $B$.

**Definition 6.2**

The value of $\lambda$ and the vector $V$ are called "the eigen value of the matrix $B$" respectively "the eigen vector of the matrix $B$" if they satisfy the equation

$$BV = \lambda V \,. \tag{6.28}$$

$B$ has type $(m + 2) \times (m + 2)$. We can find $m + 2$ eigen values of $B$ by solving a characteristic equation

$$\det(B - \lambda I) = 0 \tag{6.29}$$

where $I$ is a unit matrix of the same type $(m + 2) \times (m + 2)$.

Among $m + 2$ roots of (6.29) there exists the largest one. By returning to Eq. (6.28) we determine the coordinates of a corresponding eigen vector $V$. These constitute weights of the objectives taking place in the decision set $D$.

**Example 6.9**

Equation (6.29) results in a determinant equation

$$\det\begin{bmatrix} 1-\lambda & 3 & 5 & 7 & 7 \\ \frac{1}{3} & 1-\lambda & 3 & 7 & 7 \\ \frac{1}{5} & \frac{1}{3} & 1-\lambda & 7 & 7 \\ \frac{1}{7} & \frac{1}{7} & \frac{1}{7} & 1-\lambda & 3 \\ \frac{1}{7} & \frac{1}{7} & \frac{1}{7} & \frac{1}{3} & 1-\lambda \end{bmatrix} = 135\lambda^5 - 675\lambda^4 - 2172\lambda^2 - 1440\lambda - 320 = 0$$

which has only one real root $\lambda = 5.5805$. The associated eigen vector $V = (0.83215, 0.46393, 0.26609, 0.08575, 0.055586)$ is composed of components that are interpreted as the weights sought for $K_t$, $t = 1, \ldots, 5$.

The sets $K_t$, $t = 1, \ldots, 5$, already found in Ex. 6.7, are now completed by introducing their grades of importance.

Thus,

$$K_1 = 1^{0.83215}\big/a_1 + 0.5^{0.83215}\big/a_2 + 0.3^{0.83215}\big/a_3 + 0.3^{0.83215}\big/a_4 \,,$$

$$K_2 = 0.8^{0.46393}\big/a_1 + 0.5^{0.46393}\big/a_2 + 0.3^{0.46393}\big/a_3 + 0.3^{0.46393}\big/a_4 \,,$$

$$K_3 = 0.1^{0.26609}\Big/_{a_1} + 0.3^{0.26609}\Big/_{a_2} + 0.2^{0.26609}\Big/_{a_3} + 0.8^{0.26609}\Big/_{a_4},$$

$$K_4 = 0.8^{0.08575}\Big/_{a_1} + 0.7^{0.08575}\Big/_{a_2} + 0.4^{0.08575}\Big/_{a_3} + 0.8^{0.08575}\Big/_{a_4}$$

and

$$K_5 = 0.8^{0.055586}\Big/_{a_1} + 0.8^{0.055586}\Big/_{a_2} + 0.9^{0.055586}\Big/_{a_3} + 0.8^{0.055586}\Big/_{a_4}.$$

The final decision $D$ is obtained as a fuzzy set due to the recommended Eqs (6.26) and (6.27)

$$\begin{aligned}
D = {} & \min(1^{0.83215}, 0.8^{0.46393}, 0.1^{0.26609}, 0.8^{0.08575}, 0.8^{0.055586})\Big/_{a_1} + \\
& \min(0.5^{0.83215}, 0.5^{0.46393}, 0.3^{0.26609}, 0.7^{0.08575}, 0.8^{0.055586})\Big/_{a_2} + \\
& \min(0.3^{0.83215}, 0.3^{0.46393}, 0.2^{0.26609}, 0.4^{0.08575}, 0.9^{0.055586})\Big/_{a_3} + \\
& \min(0.3^{0.83215}, 0.3^{0.46393}, 0.8^{0.26609}, 0.8^{0.08575}, 0.8^{0.055586})\Big/_{a_4} = \\
& \min(1, 0.902, 0.542, 0.981, 0.987)\Big/_{a_1} + \min(0.562, 0.725, 0.726, 0.969, 0.987)\Big/_{a_2} + \\
& \min(0.367, 0.572, 0.652, 0.924, 0.994)\Big/_{a_3} + \\
& \min(0.367, 0.572, 0.942, 0.981, 0.988)\Big/_{a_4} = \\
& 0.5418\Big/_{a_1} + 0.5616\Big/_{a_2} + 0.3671\Big/_{a_3} + 0.3671\Big/_{a_4}.
\end{aligned}$$

We conclude that the curative power of considered medicines is ranked in the order $a_2 \approx a_1 \succ a_4 = a_3$. We have not only considered the effectiveness of drugs regarding their action on symptoms, but also the priority of symptoms. The importance order among the symptoms points out that the ones that should disappear first, for the reason of their harm, mostly influence the patient's mental and psychical condition.

### 6.4.3 Minimization of Regret

The action of the minimum operation in the final decision formula has provided us with a very cautious prognosis referring to the drug hierarchy. Some high values of degrees that reflect a positive effect of medicine, impact on considered symptoms and have no chance of influencing finally computed decision values. We can even say that the minimum operation acts as a filter for high values by depriving them of their power.

We try to obtain clearer results by applying another fuzzy decision-making technique known as a minimization of regret [84]. Let us prepare a new medical apparatus by reorganizing the sets previously introduced. We preserve a decision space (a space of alternatives) $A = \{a_1, ..., a_n\}$ but we complement a space of states as $X = \{x_1, x_2, ..., x_m, x_{m+1}, x_{m+2}\}$. In $X$ there are symbols possessing the following meanings: $x_1$ – the 1[st] symptom, …, $x_m$ – the $m^{\text{th}}$ symptom, $x_{m+1}$ – medicine side effects, $x_{m+2}$ – medicine price availability. We form a basic payoff matrix

$$C = \begin{array}{c} \\ a_1 \\ \vdots \\ a_i \\ \vdots \\ a_n \end{array} \begin{array}{c} x_1 \quad \cdots \quad x_t \quad \cdots \quad x_{m+2} \\ \left[ \begin{array}{ccccc} & & & & \\ & & & & \\ & & c_{it} & & \\ & & & & \\ & & & & \end{array} \right] \end{array}, \tag{6.30}$$

where $c_{it}$ is the payoff to a decision-maker if he connects $a_i$ to $x_t$, $i = 1, …, n$, $t = 1, …, m+2$.

In a continuation of the proposed approach to the choice of an optimal medicine, we first obtain the regret matrix $R$. Its components $r_{it}$ indicate the decision-maker's regret in selecting alternative $a_i$ when the state of $X$ is $x_t$. We then calculate the maximal regret for each alternative.

A procedure of selecting an optimal $a_i$ should follow some steps listed below:

1. For each $x_t$ calculate $C_t = \max\limits_{1 \le i \le n} c_{it}$.
2. For each pair $a_i$ and $x_t$ calculate $r_{it} = C_t - c_{it}$.
3. Suppose that matrix $B$ from Subsection 6.4.2 consists of $b_{tl}$, which now describe the importance scale when comparing states $x_t$ and $x_l$, $t$, $l = 1, …, m + 2$. The coordinates of this eigen vector that assists the largest in magnitude eigen value of $B$ still constitute weights $w_1, …, w_{m+2}$ assigned to states $x_1, …, x_{m+2}$ stated in $X$. The weights are involved in the computations of estimates $RT_i = w_1 r_{i1} + \cdots + w_{m+2} r_{i,m+2}$ for each $a_i$. It can be proved that the formulas derived for calculations of $RT_i$ satisfy the conditions of OWA operators [82, 86].
4. Select $a_{i*}$, such that $RT_{i*} = \min\limits_{1 \le i \le n} RT_i$.

The values $r_{it}$ constitute the entries of the matrix $R$ called the regret matrix. We shall refer to $C_t$ as the horizon under $x_t$.

**Example 6.10**

The sets $K_1$–$K_5$ found in Ex. 6.7 are now utilized as columns of the matrix $C$, determined by a table

$$C = \begin{array}{c} \\ a_1 \\ a_2 \\ a_3 \\ a_4 \end{array} \begin{array}{c} \begin{array}{ccccc} x_1 & x_2 & x_3 & x_4 & x_5 \end{array} \\ \begin{bmatrix} 1* & 0.8* & 0.1 & 0.8* & 0.8 \\ 0.5 & 0.5 & 0.3 & 0.7 & 0.8 \\ 0.3 & 0.3 & 0.2 & 0.4 & 0.9* \\ 0.3 & 0.3 & 0.8* & 0.8* & 0.8 \end{bmatrix} \end{array}$$

in which "*" points to the largest element in each column due to Step 1.

The regret matrix $R$ is computed as the next table

$$R = \begin{array}{c} \\ a_1 \\ a_2 \\ a_3 \\ a_4 \end{array} \begin{array}{c} \begin{array}{ccccc} x_1 & x_2 & x_3 & x_4 & x_5 \end{array} \\ \begin{bmatrix} 0 & 0 & 0.7 & 0 & 0.1 \\ 0.5 & 0.3 & 0.5 & 0.1 & 0.1 \\ 0.7 & 0.5 & 0.6 & 0.4 & 0 \\ 0.7 & 0.5 & 0 & 0 & 0.1 \end{bmatrix} \end{array}.$$

For $w_1 \approx 0.83$, $w_2 \approx 0.46$, $w_3 \approx 0.27$, $w_4 \approx 0.09$, $w_5 \approx 0.05$ (Ex. 6.9) the values of $RT_i$, $i = 1, \ldots, 4$, are appreciated as

$$RT_1 = 0.83 \cdot 0 + 0.46 \cdot 0 + 0.27 \cdot 0.7 + 0.09 \cdot 0 + 0.05 \cdot 0.1 = 0.194,$$
$RT_2 = 0.702$, $RT_3 = 1.009$, $RT_4 = 0.816$.

Finally, we decide the hierarchical order of drugs with respect to their curative abilities. We state them in sequence $a_1 \succ a_2 \succ a_4 \succ a_3$ that totally confirms the results obtained by the technique of unequal objectives. Moreover, we notice that the last decision is very clearly interpretable and easy to understand without special doubts. This emphasizes an advantage of applying the OWA weighted operations that prevent a loss of substantial information. The OWA operations have resulted in the simultaneous engagement of all effectiveness quantities in mean decision-making values involved in the regret model.

In Section 6.4 we have adapted Yager's theoretical fuzzy decision models in the process of extracting the best medicine from the collection of proposed remedies. The basis of the investigations has been mostly restricted to a judgment of medicinal influence on clinical symptoms that accompany the disease. By employing the factors of importance associated with decisive objectives we could strengthen their crucial power as well.

We have shown some useful fuzzy decision making models in the process of selecting the most efficacious medicine. The decision patterns should be particularly helpful in doubtful cases when we observe unequal, curative abilities of different medicines in the case of the same symptoms, or, when some specialists who make a trial of prioritizing the medicines have shared opinions in their judgments.

# 7 Approximation of Clock-like Point Sets

## 7.1 Introduction

This chapter has a theoretical character and can be studied by some medical staff researchers that seek methods of approximation of very irregular point sets. When the shape of an obtained polygon based on the point set is similar to a chain of bells, then it will be difficult to find a continuous standard curve that should approximate the polygon without making a large approximation error. The studies of some medical data give rise to the creation of polygons consisting of finite numbers of points tied together. Since the polygons are not formalized by some mathematical expressions, we suggest creating continuous functions that approximate them thoroughly in spite of their irregular shapes. To warrant a high accuracy of approximation, otherwise impossible to obtain when using standard curves, we test a continuous function composed of joined truncated $\pi$-functions or joined truncated $s$-functions.

By operating with the functions representing polygons that have unusual shapes, we attempt a classification of medical data. We adopt rough sets to assign the members to an investigated medical class even if their origin sometimes is unknown.

Since we do not possess medical data that comes from solidly accomplished investigations, we will discuss the matter of approximation and classification theoretically. Nevertheless, we hope that some scientists can find patterns of points in their research work that resemble the shapes assumed below. In this way they can find the proposed approximation method useful in possible research investigations of medical results.

## 7.2 Fitting of $\pi$-functions to Clock-like Polygons

Some examinations of the behaviour of the two variables named $X$ and $Y$, provide us with strings of values $x$ and $y$, which can be included in the pairs $(x, y)$, and treated further as the coordinates of points in the two-dimensional system. We suppose that the finite set $A$ consists of the points $(x, y)$, thus it can be illustrated as a polygon with its points joined together by segments of straight lines.

Certain experiments, in which $y \in [0, 1]$, deliver the polygon (set $A$) composed of parts looking like bells (or hills), e.g., like $A$, sketched in Fig. 7.1. The polygon,

Elisabeth Rakus-Andersson: *Fuzzy and Rough Techniques in Medical Diagnosis and Medication*,
StudFuzz **212**, 155–181 (2007)
www.springerlink.com

which ties a lot of straight-line bits, cannot constitute a piecewise interpolation of the points. There can be too many first-degree equations to make the further analysis of set $A$ efficient, and moreover, the linear interpolation is not smooth enough.

The most popular classical method of approximating applied to a set of points is known as the least-square regression with modern variants [15]. Other algorithms of approximating that we can mention, adopt such technical tools as cubic polynomials based on four points [43], tangent curves [1], free algebras [35] or weighted approximations [71].

As the counterpart of the listed procedures, we consider an approximation of multi-shapes from Fig. 7.1 by $\pi$-truncated functions used piecewise [65, 66]. The $y$-values of $\pi$ functions and the $y$-coordinates of the points constituting the elements of $A$ belong to the interval [0, 1]. The procedure forms the approximation of $A$ by truncated $\pi$-functions, and tied by pieces of straight lines if needed.

**Example 7.1**

In experimental domains of science like some medical investigations, we encounter polygons as results of accomplished observations in which the variable $Y$ is dependent on the variable $X$. We observe the behaviour of two variables $X$ and $Y$, to determine a finite set of pairs $A = \{(x, y)\}$, $x \in [0, 50]$, $y \in [0, 1]$. Suppose that an experiment delivers set $A$ resembling the polygon from Fig. 7.1

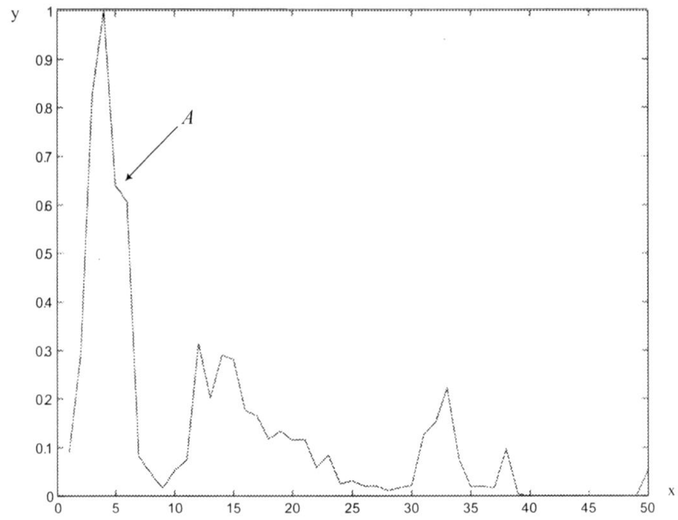


Figure 7.1: The polygon reflecting $A = \{(x, y)\}$

We will introduce "the sampled truncated $\pi$" as a split curve that approximates the polygon 7.1. This will consist of first and second degree-polynomials. The curve should follow the polygon's shape very closely to cumulate a very low error referring to deviations between the approximating curve and the polygon. We assume that a continuous function, which provides us with $y$-values corresponding to regularly chosen $x$ (not always appearing in the set of points), is more useful in the further analysis of polygons, e.g., their comparison.

We now intend to explain how to adjust a $\pi$-function to the shape of a polygon. Let us first suppose that one part $A_1$ of the obtained polygon $A$, whose shape resembles a bell, is determined by a set of pairs $(x, y)$ that represent the finite set of pairs $A_1 \subseteq A$.

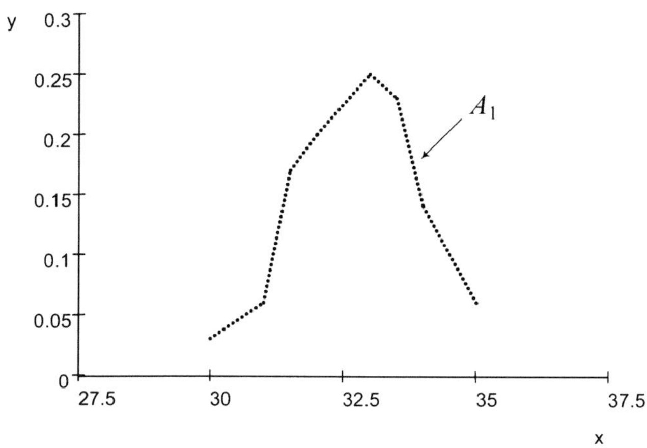


Figure 7.2: The polygon representing $A_1$

**Example 7.2**

We examine the values of pairs included in set $A_1$, which constitutes a part of $A$ presented by Fig. 7.1, over the interval (30, 35). We find that $A_1$ is determined by $A_1$ = {(30, 0.03), (31, 0.06), (31.5, 0.17), (32, 0.20), (33, 0.25), (33.5, 0.23), (34, 0.14), (35, 0.06)}. The points corresponding to the pairs given above are tied together to build the polygon $A_1$ drawn in Fig. 7.2.

To an approximation of the pattern of points from Fig. 7.2, the $\pi$-function, already inserted by (2.6) best fits because of its clock-like shape and its range constituting the interval [0, 1].

We quote the formula of $\pi$ in the fully developed form as [65, 66]

$$
y = \begin{cases}
(1)\ 0 & \text{for} \quad x < \alpha_1, \\
(2)\ 2\varepsilon\left(\dfrac{x-\alpha_1}{\gamma_1-\alpha_1}\right)^2 & \text{for} \quad \alpha_1 \le x < \beta_1, \\
(3)\ \varepsilon\left(1-2\left(\dfrac{x-\gamma_1}{\gamma_1-\alpha_1}\right)^2\right) & \text{for} \quad \beta_1 \le x < \gamma_1, \\
(4)\ \varepsilon & \text{for} \quad x = \gamma_1 = \alpha_2, \\
(5)\ \varepsilon\left(1-2\left(\dfrac{x-\alpha_2}{\gamma_2-\alpha_2}\right)^2\right) & \text{for} \quad \alpha_2 < x < \beta_2, \\
(6)\ 2\varepsilon\left(\dfrac{x-\gamma_2}{\gamma_2-\alpha_2}\right)^2 & \text{for} \quad \beta_2 \le x \le \gamma_2, \\
(7)\ 0 & \text{for} \quad x > \gamma_2.
\end{cases} \tag{7.1}
$$

The function possesses six standard parameters $\alpha_1$, $\beta_1$, $\gamma_1$, $\alpha_2$, $\beta_2$, $\gamma_2$, and it has the additional parameter $\varepsilon$, added in (7.1), which accommodates the height of the function to the real data existing in set $A_1$. The parameters $\beta_1$ and $\beta_2$ are estimated by

$$
\beta_1 = \frac{\alpha_1 + \gamma_1}{2}, \ \beta_2 = \frac{\alpha_2 + \gamma_2}{2}. \tag{7.2}
$$

**Example 7.3**

Once again we intend to recall what the $\pi$-function given by (7.1) and (7.2) looks like. If we suppose that, e.g., $\alpha_1 = 30$, $\gamma_1 = \alpha_2 = 32.5$, $\gamma_2 = 35$, and $\varepsilon = 0.25$ then $\beta_1 = \dfrac{30+32.5}{2} = 31.25$, $\beta_2 = \dfrac{32.5+35}{2} = 33.75$ and the function will have the graph depicted in Fig. 7.3.

The pairs in set $A_1$ from Ex. 7.2 have no $y$-coordinates equal to zero and that means that the values of $\alpha_1$, and $\gamma_2$ in the $\pi$-function, which is expected to approximate $A_1$, are unknown. By accepting the value of $\varepsilon$ as the largest $y$-coordinate in $A_1$, corresponding to the $x$-coordinate taken as $\gamma_1 = \alpha_2$, we reconstruct the values of remaining parameters $\alpha_1$, $\gamma_2$ according to the following patterns:

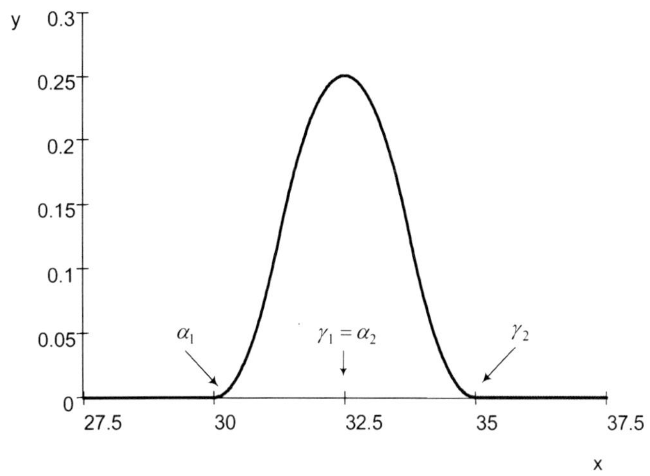


Figure 7.3: The $\pi$-function for $\alpha_1 = 30$, $\gamma_1 = \alpha_2 = 32.5$, $\gamma_2 = 35$ and $\varepsilon = 0.25$

**Case of $\alpha_1$**

Denote by $A_1(X)$ all $x$-values that belong to $n$ points from $A_1$. If the pair $(x_{\min}, y(x_{\min}))$ begins set $A_1$, which means that $x_{\min} = \min_{1 \le k \le n} x_k, x_k \in A_1(X)$ and $y(x_{\min})$ is the corresponding $y$-value to $x_{\min}$, then

a) $\alpha_1 = \dfrac{x_{\min} - \gamma_1 \sqrt{\frac{y(x_{\min})}{2\varepsilon}}}{1 - \sqrt{\frac{y(x_{\min})}{2\varepsilon}}}$ for $y(x_{\min}) < \dfrac{\varepsilon}{2}$. The value of $\alpha_1$ is computed from the equality $2\varepsilon \left( \dfrac{x_{\min} - \alpha_1}{\gamma_1 - \alpha_1} \right)^2 = y(x_{\min})$. This case entails the changes in (7.1) in accordance with

$$y = \begin{cases} (1) & 0 & \text{for} \quad x < x_{\min}, \\ (2) & 2\varepsilon \left( \dfrac{x - \alpha_1}{\gamma_1 - \alpha_1} \right)^2 & \text{for} \quad x_{\min} \le x < \beta_1, \\ (3)-(7) & \text{without changes.} & \end{cases} \tag{7.3}$$

b) $\alpha_1 = \gamma_1 - \dfrac{\gamma_1 - x_{\min}}{\sqrt{\frac{\varepsilon - y(x_{\min})}{2\varepsilon}}}$ for $y(x_{\min}) \ge \dfrac{\varepsilon}{2}$. The result is obtained from a connection

$\varepsilon\left(1-2\left(\frac{x_{\min}-\gamma_1}{\gamma_1-\alpha_1}\right)^2\right)=y(x_{\min})$. Then the $\pi(x)$ formula appears as

$$y=\begin{cases}(1)-(2) & 0 & \text{for} \quad x<x_{\min}, \\ (3) & \varepsilon\left(1-2\left(\dfrac{x-\gamma_1}{\gamma_1-\alpha_1}\right)^2\right) & \text{for} \quad x_{\min}\le x<\gamma_1, \\ (4)-(7) & \text{without changes.} & \end{cases} \tag{7.4}$$

**Case of $\gamma_2$**

The pair $(x_{\max}, y(x_{\max}))$ is the last pair in set $A_1$, which is associated with the formula $x_{\max} = \max\limits_{1\le k\le n} x_k, x_k \in A_1(X)$. Hence

c) $\gamma_2=\dfrac{x_{\max}-\alpha_2\sqrt{\frac{y(x_{\max})}{2\varepsilon}}}{1-\sqrt{\frac{y(x_{\max})}{2\varepsilon}}}$ is evaluated from part $2\varepsilon\left(\frac{x_{\max}-\gamma_2}{\gamma_2-\alpha_2}\right)^2=y(x_{\max})$ for

$y(x_{\max})<\frac{\varepsilon}{2}$. We thus suggest the following changes in (7.1) to adapt it to the new assumptions

$$y=\begin{cases}(1)-(5) & \text{without changes} & \\ (6) & 2\varepsilon\left(\dfrac{x-\gamma_2}{\gamma_2-\alpha_2}\right)^2 & \text{for} \quad \beta_2\le x<x_{\max}, \\ (7) & 0 & \text{for} \quad x\ge x_{\max}. \end{cases} \tag{7.5}$$

d) $\gamma_2=\alpha_2+\dfrac{x_{\max}-\alpha_2}{\sqrt{\frac{\varepsilon-y(x_{\max})}{2\varepsilon}}}$ for $y(x_{\max})\ge\frac{\varepsilon}{2}$ when taking into consideration the association $\varepsilon\left(1-2\left(\frac{x_{\max}-\alpha_2}{\gamma_2-\alpha_2}\right)^2\right)=y(x_{\max})$. We adjust the $\pi(x)$ formula as

$$y=\begin{cases}(1)-(4) & \text{without changes} & \\ (5) & \varepsilon\left(1-2\left(\dfrac{x-\alpha_2}{\gamma_2-\alpha_2}\right)^2\right) & \text{for} \quad \alpha_2\le x<x_{\max}, \\ (6)-(7) & 0 & \text{for} \quad x\ge x_{\max}. \end{cases} \tag{7.6}$$

The modified $\pi$ constitutes a segment of the classical $\pi$-function, therefore we will name it a truncated $\pi$-function.

We select the minimal and the maximal $x$-values as well as the maximal $y$-value existing in set $A_1$ by examining the slope of $A_1$. Equations (7.3)–(7.6) are applied to computations of unknown parameters $\alpha_1$ and $\gamma_2$. The point in which the $y$-coordinate takes the $\varepsilon$-value and the $x$-coordinate – the $\alpha_2 = \gamma_1$ value, belongs both to the polygon and the function $\pi$. In spite of reconstructing the values of $\alpha_1$ and $\gamma_2$, the approximating function is not intersected by the $x$-axis. The domain of $\pi$ begins with $A_1(X)$'s minimal $x$-value and is ended by the maximal $x$ value in $A_1(X)$. This warrants that the polygon and the curve lie very close to each other.

**Example 7.4**

The adjustments, accomplished for the data describing $A_1$ from Ex. 7.2, should be made by applying both (7.3) and (7.5). We determine $x_{\min} = 30$, $x_{\max} = 35$ and $\varepsilon = 0.25$. The $x$-coordinate associated with the largest $y$-value in $A_1$ accepted as $\varepsilon$ is equal to $\gamma_1 = \alpha_2 = 33$. Since $y(x_{\min}) = 0.03$ satisfies the condition $y(x_{\min}) < \frac{\varepsilon}{2}$, then we will compute the lacking value of the function parameter $\alpha_1$ as

$$\alpha_1 = \frac{x_{\min} - \gamma_1\sqrt{\frac{y(x_{\min})}{2\varepsilon}}}{1-\sqrt{\frac{y(x_{\min})}{2\varepsilon}}} = \frac{30-33\sqrt{\frac{0.03}{2\cdot 0.25}}}{1-\sqrt{\frac{0.03}{2\cdot 0.25}}} = 29.0278\,.$$

The value of $y(x_{\max}) = 0.06$ fulfils $y(x_{\max}) < \frac{\varepsilon}{2}$ and we will generate

$$\gamma_2 = \frac{x_{\max} - \alpha_2\sqrt{\frac{y(x_{\max})}{2\varepsilon}}}{1-\sqrt{\frac{y(x_{\max})}{2\varepsilon}}} = \frac{35-33\sqrt{\frac{0.06}{2\cdot 0.25}}}{1-\sqrt{\frac{0.06}{2\cdot 0.25}}} = 36.0918\,.$$

With $\beta_1 = 31.0139$ and $\beta_2 = 34.5459$ as the complementary parameters of the truncated $\pi_1$-function accommodated to the set $A_1$, now has a full expansion as

$$y = \begin{cases} 0.25\cdot 2\left(\dfrac{x-29.0278}{33-29.0278}\right)^2 & \text{for} \quad 30 \le x < 31.0139, \\ 0.25\left(1-2\left(\dfrac{x-33}{33-29.0278}\right)^2\right) & \text{for} \quad 31.0139 \le x < 33, \\ 0.25 & \text{for} \quad x = 33, \\ 0.25\left(1-2\left(\dfrac{x-33}{36.0918-33}\right)^2\right) & \text{for} \quad 33 < x < 34.5459, \\ 0.25\cdot 2\left(\dfrac{x-36.0918}{36.0918-33}\right)^2 & \text{for} \quad 34.5459 \le x \le 35. \end{cases}$$

Figure 7.4 shows the total effects of evaluating the finite point set $A_1$ by a continuous function $\pi_1(x)$ possessing the reconstructed parameters $\alpha_1 = 29.0278$, $\gamma_2 = 36.0918$ and $\varepsilon = 0.25$.

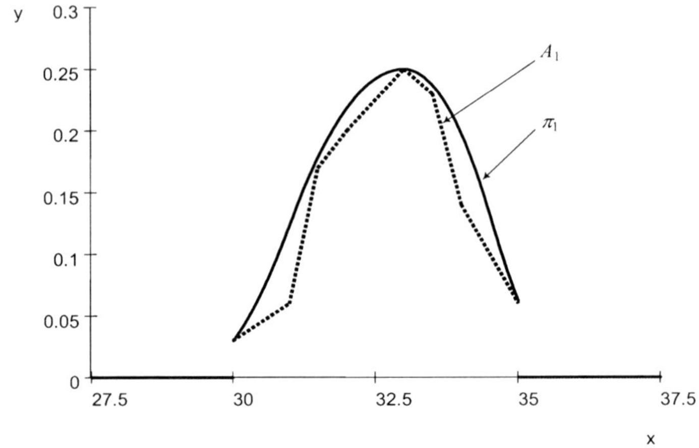


Figure 7.4: The approximation of $A_1$ by the truncated $\pi$-function

To get the collection of split definitions covering the total $x$-interval of $A$, we divide $A$'s $x$-interval in subintervals according to the magnitude of $y$-values. If the points included in $A$ create structures that resemble bells, then the $y$-coordinates of the points should be arranged in ascending order until they reach the maximal value. Afterwards the $y$-values ought to be placed in a sequence that is characterized by their descending order. If the order is ascending again, we should design a new interval for another truncated $\pi$ function. A straight line will tie the borders of two adjacent $\pi$ curves.

**Example 7.5**

Let us add the next set of points to $A_1$, known from Ex. 7.2, over the interval [35, 39] to introduce $A^* = \{(30, 0.03), (31, 0.06), (31.5, 0.17), (32, 0.20), (33, 0.25), (33.5, 0.23), (34, 0.14), (35, 0.06), (36.5, 0.07), (36.9, 0.08), (37.2, 0.09), (38, 0.1), (38.2, 0.08), (38.5, 0.06), (38.7, 0.04), (39, 0.02)\}$. We study the slopes of the polygon $A^*$ by examining the inequality relations among the $y$-values as $0.03 < 0.06 < 0.17 < 0.20 < 0.25 > 0.23 > 0.14 > 0.06 < 0.07 < 0.08 < 0.09 < 0.1 > 0.08 > 0.06 > 0.04 > 0.02$. The $y$-values form two clock shapes over [30, 35] and [36.5, 39]. We thus recognize two point sets $A_1 = \{(30, 0.03), (31, 0.06), (31.5, 0.17), (32, 0.20), (33, 0.25), (33.5, 0.23), (34, 0.14), (35, 0.06)\}$ and $A_2 = \{(36.5, 0.07), (36.9, 0.08), (37.2, 0.09), (38, 0.1), (38.2, 0.08), (38.5, 0.06), (38.7, 0.04), (39, 0.02)\}$ in $A^*$. The approximation of $A_1$ has already been accomplished in Ex. 7.4. By repeating the steps of the procedure from Ex. 7.4, we decide the unknown parameters of $\pi_2$ that intends to approximate $A_2$. We find $x_{min} = 36.5$, $x_{max} = 39$ and $\varepsilon$

= 0.1. The $x$-coordinate corresponding to $\varepsilon$ has a value of $\gamma_1 = \alpha_2 = 38$. We check that $y(x_{\min}) = 0.07$ fits for $y(x_{\min}) > \frac{\varepsilon}{2}$, which generates the parameter $\alpha_1$ as $\alpha_1 = \gamma_1 - \frac{\gamma_1 - x_{\min}}{\sqrt{\frac{\varepsilon - y(x_{\min})}{2\varepsilon}}} = 38 - \frac{38 - 36.5}{\sqrt{\frac{0.1-0.07}{2 \cdot 0.1}}} = 34.124$. The value of $y(x_{\max}) = 0.02$, however, satisfies the constraint $y(x_{\max}) < \frac{\varepsilon}{2}$; therefore we will calculate the value of $\gamma_2 = \frac{x_{\max} - \alpha_2\sqrt{\frac{y(x_{\max})}{2\varepsilon}}}{1 - \sqrt{\frac{y(x_{\max})}{2\varepsilon}}} = \frac{39 - 38\sqrt{\frac{0.02}{2 \cdot 0.1}}}{1 - \sqrt{\frac{0.02}{2 \cdot 0.1}}} = 39.449$. The additional parameters $\beta_1$ = 36.062 and $\beta_2 = 38.724$ are also included in the truncated $\pi_2$-function that matches set $A_2$ in accordance with (7.4) and (7.5).

For two points $(x_1, y_1) = (35, 0.06)$ that ends $A_1$ and $(x_2, y_2) = (36.5, 0.07)$ which begins $A_2$, we apply the equation of a straight line $y = kx + l$ in order to tie them together.

The coefficients $k$ and $l$ are computed by the formulas

$$k = \frac{y_2 - y_1}{x_2 - x_1} = \frac{0.07 - 0.06}{36.5 - 35} = 0.0067 \text{ and } l = y_2 - x_2\frac{y_2 - y_1}{x_2 - x_1} =$$

$$0.07 - 36.5\frac{0.07 - 0.06}{36.5 - 35} = -0.1746 .$$

Figure 7.5 presents the graphs of $A_1$ and $A_2$ as well as the approximating curves $\pi_1$ and $\pi_2$ joined by $y = 0.0067x - 0.1746$.

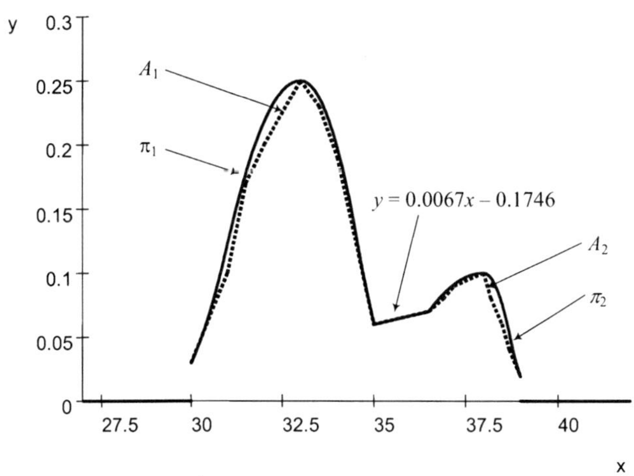


Figure 7.5: The approximation of $A^*$ by truncated $\pi$ functions

If we add the function created for $A_1$ in Ex. 7.4 to

$$y = \begin{cases} 0.0067x - 0.1746 & \text{for} \quad 35 \le x < 36.5, \\ 0.1\left(1 - 2\left(\dfrac{x-38}{38-34.124}\right)^2\right) & \text{for} \quad 36.5 \le x < 38, \\ 0.1\left(1 - 2\left(\dfrac{x-38}{39.449-38}\right)^2\right) & \text{for} \quad 38 \le x < 38.724, \\ 0.1\left(2\left(\dfrac{x-39.449}{39.449-38}\right)^2\right) & \text{for} \quad 38.724 \le x \le 39, \end{cases}$$

then we will obtain the total approximating function for $A^*$.

By using the same procedure to all "bells" visible in $A$ in Fig. 7.1, we obtain other functions of the $\pi$ type. We join the functions by inserting equations of straight lines to plot a full, continuous curve $\pi(x)$ approximating $A$ entirely.

Since we adapt several $\pi$ functions to truncated forms, then we will call a sampled approximation "sampled, truncated $\pi$".

**Example 7.6**

Figure 7.1 is an example of the point set, which delivers an irregular polygon $A = \{(x, y)\}$. The polygon is composed of segments of straight lines that tie $(x, y)$ together. Figure 7.6 gives the approximation of the shape's image from Fig. 7.1, by a collection of truncated $\pi$ functions joined together by pieces of lines to guarantee continuity of the approximating function.

It is worth noticing that the collective error that measures the deviations of $\pi$ from $A$ is not large and that is very important for the approximation of a composed polygon consisting of many "bells".

A number of split functions that are included in the sampled definition of $\pi(x)$ is substantially less than a number of linear functions that define short line pieces placed among the nodes $(x, y)$ in the polygon $A$. One $\pi$ segment can surround a great many pairs $(x, y)$. This reduces the number of piecewise definitions and the number of subintervals in the "sampled truncated $\pi$". By introducing $\pi$ we simplify a collective definition of the function approximating $A$ when comparing it to the linear parts taking place in the interpolation of $A$. This property of $\pi$ should be regarded as its advantage.

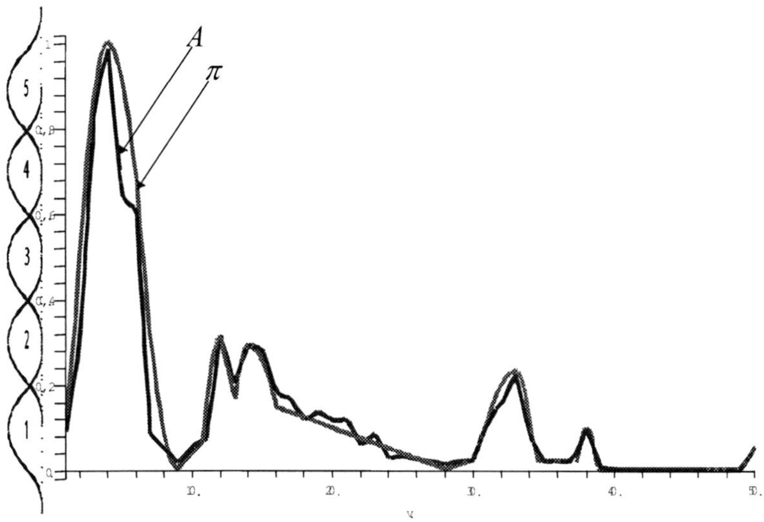


Figure 7.6: The sampled $\pi$ in the approximation of $A$

## 7.3 Rough Sets in Classifying of Clock-like Polygons

In order to include the unknown sets of the $A$ type within classes already possessing the declared members, we apply some elements of rough set theory [50, 51, 52, 53] that have already proven useful in the process of a disease classification.

The $y$-axis in Fig. 7.6 is divided in five regions. We would like to assign codes associated with the subintervals of the same length created for the $y$-values. Some scientists have a custom of applying fuzzy sets with their membership functions to accomplish the determination of interval borders [50]. Anyhow, we do not want to engage new elements of fuzzy set theory in this chapter, we only want to announce another possibility of finding the boundaries for the named intervals by drawing five membership functions along the $y$-axis in Fig. 7.6. Independently of the method, we list intervals of the $y$-variable and associated with them codes in Table 7.1.

Each considered point set has an envelope created by a continuous function that approximates it. When regarding any value placed on the $x$-axis we are capable of establishing the association between the $x$-value and the code. To achieve this we should first compute the $\pi(x)$ value and then place it in the appropriate interval from Table 7.1. We thus accept the set $A = \{(x, y)\} \approx \{(x, \pi(x))\} = \{(x, code(x)\}$, where $code(x)$ is the code of the $\pi(x)$ interval.

Table 7.1: The relationship between $y$-values and codes

| Interval of $y$-values | Code |
|---|---|
| (0.0, 0.2) | 1 |
| (0.2, 0.4) | 2 |
| (0.4, 0.6) | 3 |
| (0.6, 0.8) | 4 |
| (0.8, 1.0) | 5 |

Let us introduce a universe set $U=\{A_1, \ldots, A_n\}$ composed of clock-like polygons. Assume that some of them are members of class "Class 1", while the others have an unknown membership or belong to a different class other than "Class 1". Our purpose is to assign membership degrees to all polygons from $U$ in order to classify them within "Class 1".

The objects of $U$ are determined by two groups of attributes, so called condition and decision attributes, presented by the sets $B$ and $D$ respectively. We assume that set $B$ consists of $m$ chosen $x$-sizes $x_j$, mapped into a set of values $code_{A_i}(x_j)$, $i = 1, \ldots, n, j = 1, \ldots, m$. The codes are equal to the integers 1, 2, 3, 4, 5. Set $D$ has an attribute stated as "the membership of a polygon in "Class 1"", where the membership is expressed as "*yes*", "*no*" and "*unknown*".

The triple $I = (U, B, D)$ forms the decision table that constitutes a data basis for an equivalence relation $I(B)$ called the indiscernibility relation and defined by the relationship

$$I(B) = \left\{(A_i, A_k) : code_{A_i}(x_j) = code_{A_k}(x_j)\right\} \quad \textit{for each size } x_j, \tag{7.7}$$

where $j = 1, 2, \ldots, m, i, k = 1, 2, \ldots, n$.

We find the equivalence classes of the relation $I(B)$, i.e., the blocks $IB(A_i)$ as the sets

$$IB(A_i) = \{A_k : (A_i, A_k) \in I(B)\}. \tag{7.8}$$

By following a general rough set procedure we create a set $X = \{A_i :$ membership "*yes*" to "Class 1" is assigned$\}$.

The first decision set (the lower approximation of $X$)

$$B_*(X) = \{A_i : IB(A_i) \subseteq X\} \tag{7.9}$$

reveals the polygons which surely match "Class 1".

The other decision set (the upper approximation of $X$)

$$B^*(X) = \{A_i : IB(A_i) \cap X \neq 0\} \tag{7.10}$$

contains these members of $U$ that may belong to "Class 1".

The elements of a boundary set

$$B_{border}(X) = B^{*}(X) - B_{*}(X) \tag{7.11}$$

are interpreted as members of "Class 1" in a certain grade.

The membership degree of $A_i$, interpreted as a degree of being a member in "Class 1", is computed as

$$\mu_{\text{"Class 1"}}(A_i) = \frac{|X \cap IB(A_i)|}{|IB(A_i)|}. \tag{7.12}$$

**Example 7.7**

We collect the data concerning six point sets $A_1$–$A_6$ and approximate the obtained polygons by "sampled truncated $\pi$" $\pi_1$–$\pi_6$ as shown in Fig. 7.7. The continuous and smooth curves replace sharp polygons to give access to every pair $(x, y)$ over the common $x$-interval under consideration.

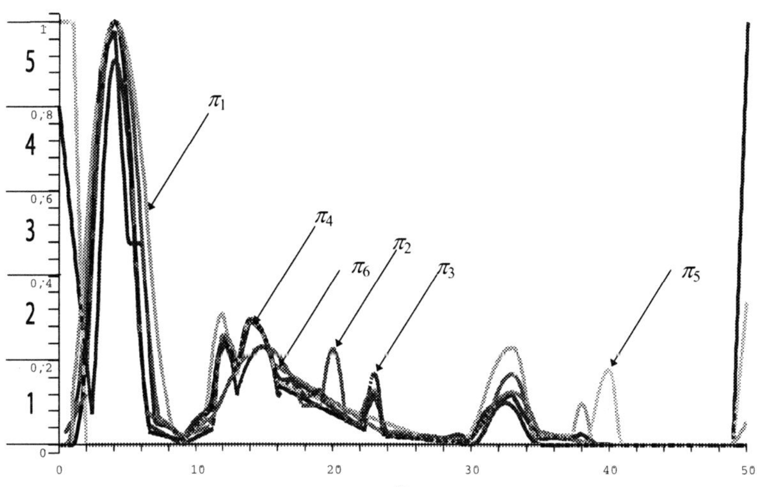


Figure 7.7: $\pi_1$–$\pi_6$ in approximation of polygons $A_1$–$A_6$

We state $U = \{A_1, A_2, A_3, A_4, A_5, A_6\}$.

The decision table $I = (U, B, D)$, made for the condition (codes 1, 2, 3, 4, 5) and decision (*yes*, *no*, *unknown*) attributes, shows the properties of members of $U$ expanded in Table 7.2.

Table 7.2: The decision table $I = (U, B, D)$ of clock-like polygons $A_1$–$A_6$

| $A_i \backslash x_j$ | 0 | 4 | 8 | 12 | 16 | 20 | 24 | 28 | "Class 1" |
|---|---|---|---|---|---|---|---|---|---|
| $A_1$ | 1 | 5 | 1 | 2 | 1 | 1 | 1 | 1 | *yes* |
| $A_2$ | 1 | 5 | 1 | 1 | 1 | 2 | 1 | 1 | *yes* |
| $A_3$ | 5 | 5 | 1 | 2 | 1 | 1 | 1 | 1 | *yes* |
| $A_4$ | 1 | 5 | 1 | 2 | 1 | 1 | 1 | 1 | *yes* |
| $A_5$ | 5 | 1 | 1 | 1 | 1 | 1 | 1 | 1 | *no* |
| $A_6$ | 1 | 5 | 1 | 2 | 1 | 1 | 1 | 1 | *unknown* |

The equivalence relation $I(B)$ is formed by a set of pairs

$$I(B) = \{(A_1, A_1), (A_2, A_2), (A_3, A_3), (A_4, A_4), (A_5, A_5), (A_6, A_6), (A_4, A_6), (A_6, A_4)\}.$$

The equivalence classes of $I(B)$ are created as the sets

$$IB(A_1) = \{A_1\},\ IB(A_2) = \{A_2\},\ IB(A_3) = \{A_3\},\ IB(A_4) = \{A_4, A_6\},\ IB(A_5) = \{A_5\},$$
$$IB(A_6) = \{A_6, A_4\}$$

according to (7.8).

The semantic value of the decision attribute "Class 1" = "*yes*" generates set $X = \{A_1, A_2, A_3, A_4\}$ that in turn is an essential factor implementing the sets $B_*(X) = \{A_1, A_2, A_3\}$, $B^*(X) = \{A_1, A_2, A_3, A_4, A_6\}$ and $B_{border}(X) = \{A_4, A_6\}$.

The polygon membership degrees whose sizes confirm the membership in "Class 1" are obtained as

$$\mu_{"Class\ 1"}(A_1) = 1,\ \mu_{"Class\ 1"}(A_2) = 1,\ \mu_{"Class\ 1"}(A_3) = 1,\ \mu_{"Class\ 1"}(A_4) = \frac{1}{2},$$

$$\mu_{"Class\ 1"}(A_5) = 0,\ \mu_{"Class\ 1"}(A_6) = \frac{1}{2}.$$

We can assume that $A_1$, $A_2$ and $A_3$ are the true members of "Class 1" in $U$ while $A_4$ and $A_6$ may belong to the investigated class to certain degrees. We can also notice that $A_6$ affects a status of $A_4$ negatively, and on the contrary, we can see that $A_4$ upgrades the importance of $A_6$ in the considered class "Class 1".

## 7.4 *s*-functions in Fitting to Letter-shaped Polygons

As effects of some experiments, in which $y \in [-1, 1]$, we obtain polygons (sets $A$) composed of parts looking like bells or even half-bells that lie over and under the $x$-axis.

**Example 7.8**

Consider the polygon $A$ sketched in Fig. 7.8.

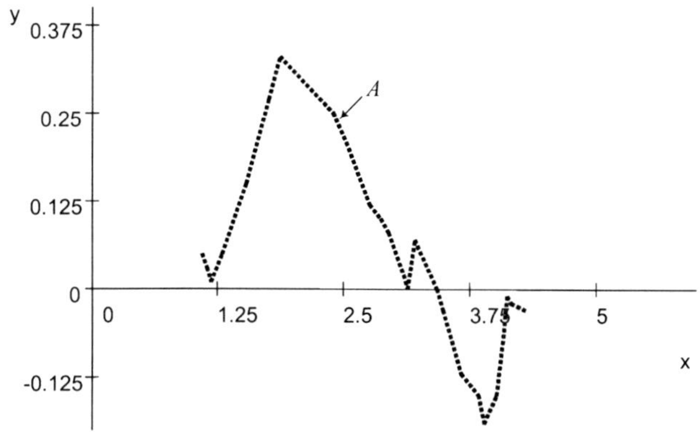


Figure 7.8: The example of a letter-shaped polygon reflecting $A = \{(x, y)\}$

We assume an approximation of multi-shapes from Fig. 7.8 by $s$-truncated functions used piecewise as another approach to the numerical problem of a smooth curve fitting to point sets. Since we recognize half-bells as dominant shapes in $A$, then we should prefer adopting the appearance of the $s$-functions as approximating segments. "The sampled truncated $s$", as we call an entire approximation curve, consists of first and second degree-polynomials. This would follow the polygon's shape very closely and results in cumulating very low error, measuring deviations between the approximating curve and the polygon.

Let us suppose that the $y$-values of curves, that are similar in shape to the set depicted in Fig. 7.8, are important indicators in the further classification process of the curves. These can resemble some letters, e.g., $N$, $W$, or $M$, and can occur in different places along the $x$-axis. In order to assign the curves to proper classes denoted by $N$, $W$ or $M$, we should compare their $y$-coordinates. It is not possible if the curves are scattered in different segments of the $x$-axis. To make the curves comparable, we should move them over the interval [0, 1].

The approach to approximation of irregular polygons presented below constitutes a solution [65, 66, 67] that differs from other modern procedures of seeking approximation curves [1, 15, 35, 43, 71].

We discover that the $x$-values of pairs included in $A$ belong to interval $[x_{\min}(A), x_{\max}(A)]$, in which $x_{\min}(A)$ is the smallest and $x_{\max}(A)$ is the largest $x$-value in $A$. In the next step we divide the whole $x$-interval into subintervals $[x_{\min(A_j)}, x_{\max(A_j)}]$, where $A_j$, $j = 1, 2, \ldots, Q$, are parts of $A$. In parts $A_j$ we can experience either the growth or the decrease of the $y$-values corresponding to these perience either the growth or the decrease of the $y$-values corresponding to these $x$ that are placed between the borders $x_{\min(A_j)}$ and $x_{\max(A_j)}$ functioning as the smallest, and respectively, the largest value of $x$ in $A_j$. $S$-functions or segments of straight lines attached to two adjacent $s$-curves approximate the $A_j$ components.

**Example 7.9**

The pairs, which create the polygon depicted in Fig. 7.8, are the members of $A$ = {(1.1, 0.05), (1.15, 0.03), (1.19, 0.01), (1.3, 0.05), (1.54, 0.15), (1.76, 0.27), (1.87, 0.33), (2.4, 0.25), (2.55, 0.2), (2.76, 0.12), (2.87, 0.1), (2.96, 0.08), (3.1, 0.02), (3.14, 0), (3.21, 0.07), (3.48, 0), (3.49, –0.03), (3.67, –0.12), (3.84, –0.15), (3.9, –0.19), (4.02, –0.15), (4.09, –0.06), (4.12, –0.01), (4.16, –0.02), (4.3, –0.03)}. By measuring the direction of changes in the $y$-values, which point out extreme nodes in $A$'s shape, we consider the subintervals [1.1, 1.19], [1.19, 1.87], [1.87, 3,14], [3.14, 3.21], [3.21, 3.43], [3.43, 3.9], [3.9, 4.12], [4.12, 4.3]. Over the intervals either $s$-functions or straight lines will be applied as approximation tools.

The $s$-function with the standard parameters $\alpha$, $\beta$, $\gamma$ and an additional parameter $\varepsilon$, introduced by (2.5) and modified by the equation

$$y = s(x,\alpha,\beta,\gamma,\varepsilon) = \begin{cases} (1) \quad \varepsilon\left(2\left(\dfrac{x-\alpha}{\gamma-\alpha}\right)^2\right) & \text{for} \quad \alpha \le x < \beta, \\ (2) \quad \varepsilon\left(1-2\left(\dfrac{x-\gamma}{\gamma-\alpha}\right)^2\right) & \text{for} \quad \beta \le x \le \gamma, \end{cases} \tag{7.13}$$

where $\beta = \dfrac{\alpha+\gamma}{2}$, is suitable for the occurrences of "half-bells" $A_j$. Since the $y$-values of the classical $s$ belong to the interval [0, 1] (–$s$ has its $y$-values in [–1, 0]) then we should insert an additional parameter $\varepsilon$ in (7.13) to accommodate a height of the function to the data existing in the set $A_j$, $j$ = 1, 2, ..., $Q$. We have already introduced the partition of $A$ by means of subsets $A_j$, looking like "half-bells", then we should denote each $s$-function that approximates $A_j$ by $s_{A_j}(x,\alpha_{A_j},\beta_{A_j},\gamma_{A_j},\varepsilon_{A_j})$.

We now discuss different cases of $A_j$'s approximation that is dependent on the sizes of $y$-coordinates in the set $A_j$.

Let us assume that the values of the $y$-coordinates in $A_j$ associated with the $x$-values belonging to $\lfloor x_{\min(A_j)}, x_{\max(A_j)} \rfloor$ appear in the ascending order, and let us notice that no $y$-coordinate is equal to zero. The pair $(x_{\min(A_j)}, y(x_{\min(A_j)}))$ (( $y(x_{\min(A_j)})$ corresponds to $x_{\min(A_j)}$) begins the set $A_j$ but we cannot identify $x_{\min(A_j)}$ as $\alpha_{A_j}$. Thus, the value of $\alpha_{A_j}$ in the $s_{A_j}$-function, expected to approximate $A_j$, is unknown. To find $\alpha_{A_j}$ we, at first, accept the value of $\varepsilon_{A_j}$ as the largest $y$-coordinate in $A_j$ associated with the $x$-coordinate $\gamma_{A_j}$. We can now reconstruct the value of the remaining parameter $\alpha_{A_j}$ according to patterns that are almost identical with "Case of $\alpha_1$" already discussed for $\pi$-functions:

a) $\alpha_{A_j} = \dfrac{x_{\min(A_j)} - \gamma_{A_j}\sqrt{\dfrac{y(x_{\min(A_j)})}{2\varepsilon_{A_j}}}}{1-\sqrt{\dfrac{y(x_{\min(A_j)})}{2\varepsilon_{A_j}}}}$ for $y(x_{\min(A_j)}) < \dfrac{\varepsilon_{A_j}}{2}$. It changes (7.13) as

$$y = \begin{cases} (1) & \varepsilon_{A_i}\left(2\left(\dfrac{x-\alpha_{A_j}}{\gamma_{A_j}-\alpha_{A_j}}\right)^2\right) & \text{for} & x_{\min(A_j)} \le x < \beta_{A_j}, \\ (2) & \varepsilon_{A_i}\left(1-2\left(\dfrac{x-\gamma_{A_j}}{\gamma_{A_j}-\alpha_{A_j}}\right)^2\right) & \text{for} & \beta_{A_j} \le x < \gamma_{A_j}. \end{cases} \tag{7.14}$$

b) $\alpha_{A_j} = \gamma_{A_j} - \dfrac{\gamma_{A_j} - x_{\min(A_j)}}{\sqrt{\dfrac{\varepsilon_{A_j} - y(x_{\min(A_j)})}{2\varepsilon_{A_j}}}}$ for $y(x_{\min(A_j)}) \ge \dfrac{\varepsilon_{A_j}}{2}$. The $s_{A_j}(x)$ formula appears as

$$y = \begin{cases} (1) & 0 & \text{for} & x < x_{\min(A_j)}, \\ (2) & \varepsilon_{A_j}\left(1-2\left(\dfrac{x-\gamma_{A_j}}{\gamma_{A_j}-\alpha_{A_j}}\right)^2\right) & \text{for} & x_{\min(A_j)} \le x \le \gamma_{A_j}. \end{cases} \tag{7.15}$$

It happens that the position of pairs in the set $A_j$ introduces the descending order among points with respect to the $y$-coordinate values. We assume that none of them is equal to zero. The pair $(x_{\max(A_j)}, y(x_{\max(A_j)}))$ will end the set $A_j$, but $x_{\max(A_j)} \neq \gamma_{A_j}$. Let us assign the largest value of $y$ in $A_j$, regarded as $\varepsilon_{A_j}$, to the $x$-coordinate $x_{\min(A_j)} = \alpha_{A_j}$. Then it is possible to restore the missing value of $\gamma_{A_j}$, which is one of the parameters included in function $1 - s_{A_j}(x, \alpha_{A_j}, \beta_{A_j}, \gamma_{A_j}, \varepsilon_{A_j})$ applied to approximate $A_j$.

We make the following distinction between two different cases of adjusting the parameter $\gamma_{A_j}$ to the data set $A_j$:

c) $\gamma_{A_j} = \dfrac{x_{\max(A_j)} - \alpha_{A_j}\sqrt{\dfrac{y(x_{\max(A_j)})}{2\varepsilon_{A_j}}}}{1-\sqrt{\dfrac{y(x_{\max(A_j)})}{2\varepsilon_{A_j}}}}$ for $y(x_{\max(A_j)}) < \dfrac{\varepsilon_{A_j}}{2}$. We suggest the following changes in (7.13) to adapt it to the new assumptions

$$y = \begin{cases} (1) \quad \varepsilon_{A_j}\left(1-2\left(\dfrac{x-\alpha_{A_j}}{\gamma_{A_j}-\alpha_{A_j}}\right)^2\right) & \text{for} \quad \alpha_{A_j} \le x < \beta_{A_j}, \\ (2) \quad \varepsilon_{A_j}\left(2\left(\dfrac{x-\gamma_{A_j}}{\gamma_{A_j}-\alpha_{A_j}}\right)^2\right) & \text{for} \quad \beta_{A_j} \le x \le x_{\max(A_j)}. \end{cases} \tag{7.16}$$

d) $\gamma_{A_j} = \alpha_{A_j} + \dfrac{x_{\max(A_j)} - \alpha_{A_j}}{\sqrt{\dfrac{\varepsilon_{A_j} - y(x_{\max(A_j)})}{2\varepsilon_{A_j}}}}$ for $y(x_{\max(A_j)}) \ge \dfrac{\varepsilon_{A_j}}{2}$. We adjust the $s_{A_j}(x)$ formula as

$$y = \begin{cases} (1) \quad \varepsilon_{A_j}\left(1-2\left(\dfrac{x-\alpha_{A_j}}{\gamma_{A_j}-\alpha_{A_j}}\right)^2\right) & \text{for} \quad \alpha_{A_j} \le x \le x_{\max(A_j)}, \\ (2) \quad 0 & \text{for} \quad x > x_{\max(A_j)}. \end{cases} \tag{7.17}$$

The $s_{A_j}$ function is a section of the classical *s*-function and therefore we will name it a truncated *s*-function. By selecting the minimal and the maximal *x*-value and the maximal *y*-value, which exist in the set $A_j$, we prepare (7.14)–(7.17) for computing the unknown parameters $\alpha_{A_j}$ or $\gamma_{A_j}$. The point, in which the *y*-coordinate takes the $\varepsilon_{A_j}$-value and the *x*-coordinate is the equal of the $\gamma_{A_j}$ value for the function $s_{A_j}(x, \alpha_{A_j}, \beta_{A_j}, \gamma_{A_j}, \varepsilon_{A_j})$, and respectively the $\alpha_{A_j}$ value for the complement $1 - s_{A_j}(x, \alpha_{A_j}, \beta_{A_j}, \gamma_{A_j}, \varepsilon_{A_j})$, is one of the vertices in *A* and it constitutes the common element of $A_j$ and the function $s_{A_j}$, $j = 1, \ldots, Q$. The total approximation $s_A$ of *A* is called "sampled truncated *s*".

To preserve the right shape of the approximating curve, it is advisable to tie two adjacent functions $s_{A_j}$, $s_{A_{j+1}}$ between the points $(x_{\max(A_j)}, y(x_{\max(A_j)}))$, $(x_{\min(A_{j+1})}, y(x_{\min(A_{j+1})}))$ by the segment of a straight line having an equation

$$y = line_{A_j}(x) = k_{A_j}x + l_{A_j} \quad \text{for} \quad x_{\max(A_j)} \le x < x_{\min(A_{j+1})}. \tag{7.18}$$

**Example 7.10**

The "sampled truncated *s*", made for the data from Ex. 7.8, is shown in Fig. 7.9.

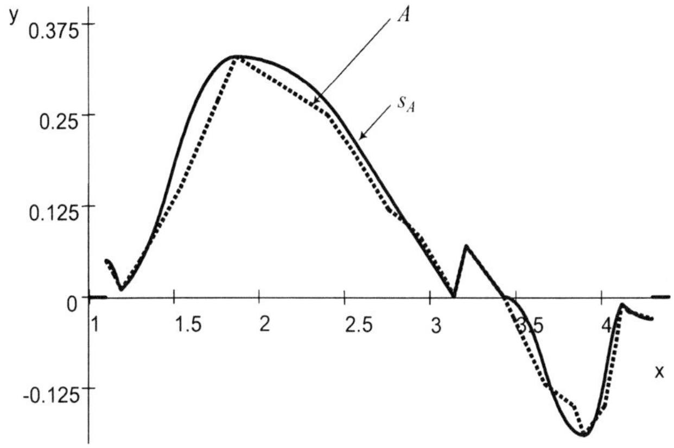


Figure 7.9: The approximation of *A* by "sampled truncated *s*"

The first set of points $A_1 \subset A$, in which the *y*-coordinates form the descending order, is placed over [1.1, 1.19] as decided in Ex. 7.9. Since no *y*-value is equal to zero we will reconstruct the value of a parameter $\gamma_{A_1} = \dfrac{1.19 - 1.1\sqrt{\frac{0.01}{2\cdot 0.05}}}{1-\sqrt{\frac{0.01}{2\cdot 0.05}}} = 1.2316$ for $\varepsilon_{A_1} = 0.05$, $\alpha_{A_1} = 1.1$, $x_{\max(A_1)} = 1.19$ and $y(x_{\max(A_1)}) = 0.01$ in accordance with c).

In the next interval $A_2$ = [1.19, 1.87] the value of $\alpha_{A_2}$ should be estimated. If we request the values of $\varepsilon_{A_2} = 0.33$, $\gamma_{A_2} = 1.87$, $x_{\min(A_2)} = 1.19$ and $y(x_{\min(A_2)}) = 0.01$ then $\alpha_{A_2} = \dfrac{1.19 - 1.87\sqrt{\frac{0.01}{2\cdot 0.33}}}{1-\sqrt{\frac{0.01}{2\cdot 0.33}}}$ =1.0945 due to a).

The formula of $s_A$ for *A* is expanded as the following split definition

$$
y = s_A(x) = \begin{cases}
0.05\left(1 - 2\left(\dfrac{x-1.1}{1.2316-1.1}\right)^2\right) & \text{for} \quad 1.1 \le x < 1.1658, \\
0.05\left(2\left(\dfrac{x-1.2316}{1.2316-1.1}\right)^2\right) & \text{for} \quad 1.1658 \le x < 1.19, \\
\vdots & \vdots \quad \vdots \\
(-0.31818)x + 1.0914 & \text{for} \quad 3.21 \le x < 3.43, \\
\vdots & \vdots \quad \vdots \\
-0.03\left(1 - 2\left(\dfrac{x-4.3}{4.3-3.9958}\right)^2\right) & \text{for} \quad 4.1479 \le x < 4.3.
\end{cases}
$$

We can prove some additional operations on the $s$-function values, e.g., $y = (s(x))^2$ or $y = (s(x))^{\frac{1}{2}}$ to match a shape of the function to the given polygon in the best way.

It is worth noticing that the total error that collects the deviations of $s_A(x)$ from $A$ is very small.

The curve created for $A$ has a particular pattern since it resembles the letter $N$. In some medical or technical problems we obtain sets of points that will be approximated by some shapes of letters, e.g., $N$, $M$ or $W$. The shapes of mentioned letters can be disturbed or vague, which makes difficult to classify them properly, i.e., we do not know exactly if we should include the curves in classes determined by $N$, $M$ and $W$. In order to ensure if a vague or unknown object can belong to the considered class or not, we accomplish a classification according to the rules of rough set theory.

If we are given several polygons then we, at the first stage, want to collect all approximated objects over a common interval [0, 1] to measure their deviations in $y$-values with respect to the same $x$ values.

**Example 7.11**

Suppose that we have obtained different shapes of the curves originating from point sets $A^1$–$A^5$. Each of them is approximated by a continuous function that consists of $s$-sections and pieces of straight lines that link the parts of $s$-functions if it is necessary. Figure 7.10 provides the polygons and the approximating functions over their original intervals along the $x$-axis. We assume the following polygon membership: $A^1$, $A^3$ and $A^5$ belong to the "$N$" class, $A^4$ is a member of the "$W$" class, while the origin of $A^2$ is unknown.

In further analysis we use only the continuous curves, also named $A^1$–$A^5$.

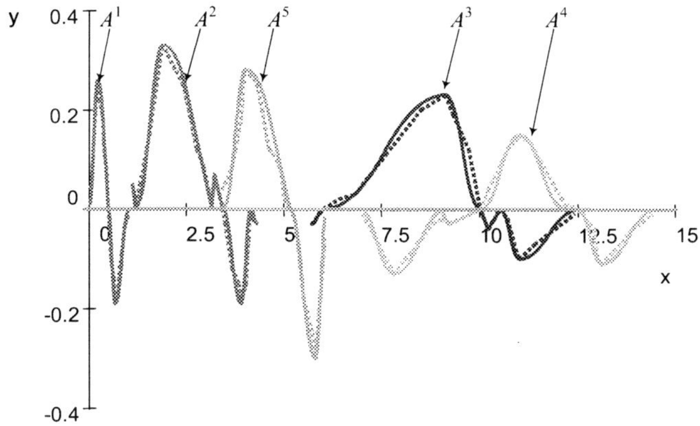


Figure 7.10: The approximated polygons $A^1$–$A^5$

To move all curves to the same starting point settled as the origin of the *x*-*y* coordinate system, we suggest the following transformations.

Suppose that the $A^i$-curve, $i = 1, \ldots, n$, is placed in the *x*-subinterval $\left[x_{\min}(A^i), x_{\max}(A^i)\right]$. We move the $j^{\text{th}}$ segment $s_{A^i_j}$, approximating the subset $A^i_j$ of $A^i$, $i = 1, \ldots, n$, $j = 1, \ldots, Q$, to a position close to the origin by introducing the formula

$$y = \begin{cases} (1)\ \varepsilon_{A^i_j}\left(2\left(\dfrac{x-(\alpha_{A^i_j}-x_{\min}(A^i))}{\gamma_{A^i_j}-\alpha_{A^i_j}}\right)^2\right) & \text{for } x_{\min(A^i_j)}-x_{\min}(A^i)\le x<\beta_{A^i_j}-x_{\min}(A^i), \\ (2)\ \varepsilon_{A^i_j}\left(1-2\left(\dfrac{x-(\gamma_{A^i_j}-x_{\min}(A^i))}{\gamma_{A^i_j}-\alpha_{A^i_j}}\right)^2\right) & \text{for } \beta_{A^i_j}-x_{\min}(A^i)\le x\le\gamma_{A^i_j}-x_{\min}(A^i). \end{cases} \tag{7.19}$$

The straight line (7.18) is transferred nearby the origin by the action of an equation

$$y = line_{A^i_j}(x) = k_{A^i_j}x + l_{A^i_j} + k_{A^i_j}\cdot x_{\min}(A^i) = K_{A^i_j}x + L_{A^i_j} \quad \text{for } x_{\max(A^i_j)} - x_{\min}(A^i) \le x < x_{\min(A^i_{j+1})} - x_{\min}(A^i) \tag{7.20}$$

**Example 7.12**

Figure 7.11 shows $A^1$–$A^5$ attached to the origin after performing (7.19) and (7.20).

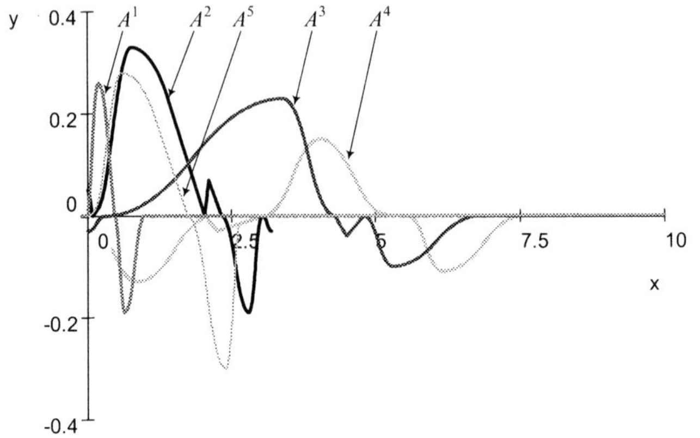


Figure 7.11: The curves $A^1$–$A^5$ with their start points at the origin

In Fig. 7.11 we recognize $A^2$ as $A$ from Ex. 7.8. We decide $x_{\min}(A^2) = 1.1$ and modify "sampled truncated $s$" for $A_2 = A$, as a function

$$y = s_{A^2}(x) = \begin{cases} 0.05\left(1 - 2\left(\dfrac{x-(1.1-1.1)}{1.2316-1.1}\right)^2\right) & \text{for} \quad 1.1-1.1 \le x < 1.1658-1.1, \\ 0.05\left(2\left(\dfrac{x-(1.2316-1.1)}{1.2316-1.1}\right)^2\right) & \text{for} \quad 1.1658-1.1 \le x < 1.19-1.1, \\ \vdots & \vdots \quad\quad \vdots \\ (-0.31818)x + 1.0914 & \\ +(-0.31818)\cdot 1.1 = & \text{for} \quad 3.21-1.1 \le x < 3.43-1.1, \\ (-0.31818)x + 0.7414 & \\ \vdots & \vdots \quad\quad \vdots \\ -0.03\left(1 - 2\left(\dfrac{x-(4.3-1.1)}{4.3-3.9958}\right)^2\right) & \text{for} \quad 4.1479-1.1 \le x < 4.3-1.1, \end{cases}$$

which displaces $A_2$'s start point to the origin.

The comparison of all curves will be successful if we can observe them at a common interval. Let us determine the interval [0, 1] as a new domain for all split-functions $A^1$–$A^n$. Each piece $s_{A^i_j}$ or $line_{A^i_j}$, $i = 1, \ldots, n$, $j = 1, \ldots, Q$, should be shrunk or enlarged proportionally to fit it for the interval [0, 1] together with other pieces.

In order to achieve the required movements of $s_j^i$ over [0, 1], we initiate the parameter $\delta_{A^i} = \dfrac{1}{x_{\max}(A^i) - x_{\min}(A^i)}$ in (7.19), which generates a new formula [49, 67]

$$y = \begin{cases} (1) \quad \varepsilon_{A_j^i}\left(2\left(\dfrac{x-(\alpha_{A_j^i} - x_{\min}(A^i))\delta_{A^i}}{(\gamma_{A_j^i} - \alpha_{A_j^i})\delta_{A^i}}\right)^2\right) \\ \text{for} \quad (x_{\min(A_j^i)} - x_{\min}(A^i))\delta_{A^i} \le x < (\beta_{A_j^i} - x_{\min}(A^i))\delta_{A^i}, \\ (2) \quad \varepsilon_{A_j^i}\left(1-2\left(\dfrac{x-(\gamma_{A_j^i} - x_{\min}(A^i))\delta_{A^i}}{(\gamma_{A_j^i} - \alpha_{A_j^i})\delta_{A^i}}\right)^2\right) \\ \text{for} \quad (\beta_{A_j^i} - x_{\min}(A^i))\delta_{A^i} \le x \le (\gamma_{A_j^i} - x_{\min}(A^i))\delta_{A^i}. \end{cases} \tag{7.21}$$

Before equipping (7.20) with the parameter $\delta_{A^i}$ we should find another form of (7.20) adapted to the range [0, 1] as [7, 67]

$$y = K_{A_j^i}x + L_{A_j^i} = \frac{x + \dfrac{L_{A_j^i}}{K_{A_j^i}}}{\dfrac{1}{K_{A_j^i}}} \quad \text{for} \quad x_{\max(A_j^i)} - x_{\min}(A^i) \le x < x_{\min(A_{j+1}^i)} - x_{\min}(A^i). \tag{7.22}$$

We can now place $\delta_{A^i}$ in (7.22) according to a pattern

$$y = \frac{x + \dfrac{L_{A_j^i}\delta_{A^i}}{K_{A_j^i}}}{\dfrac{\delta_{A^i}}{K_{A_j^i}}} \quad \text{for} \quad (x_{\max(A_j^i)} - x_{\min}(A^i))\delta_{A^i} \le x < (x_{\min(A_{j+1}^i)} - x_{\min}(A^i))\delta_{A^i}. \tag{7.23}$$

**Example 7.13**

The applications of (7.21) and (7.23) to every $s$-section and every line segment that takes place in $A^1$–$A^5$, yields the effect of collecting all curves over the $x$-domain [0, 1]. The curves $A^1$–$A^5$, lying in [0, 1], are plotted in Fig. 7.12.

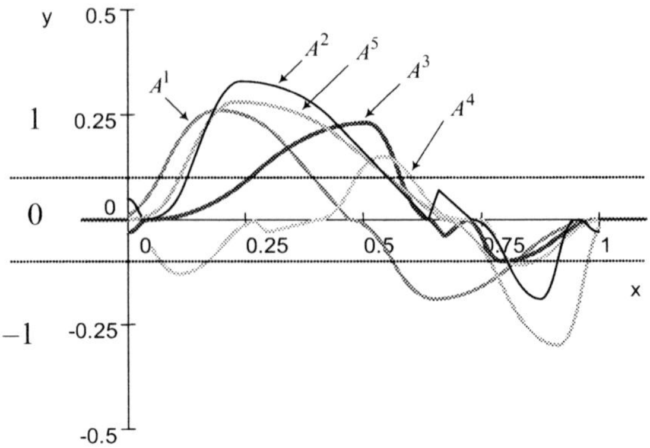


Figure 7.12: The curves $A^1$–$A^5$ over the common interval [0, 1]

After the executed transformations (7.21) and (7.23) the $y$-coordinates of $A^2$, for which $\delta_{A^2} = \dfrac{1}{4.3-1.1} \approx 0.31$, are computed as values

$$y = s_{A^2}(x) = \begin{cases} 0.05\left(1-2\left(\dfrac{x-(1.1-1.1)0.31}{(1.2316-1.1)0.31}\right)^2\right) \\ \text{for } (1.1-1.1)0.31 \le x < (1.1658-1.1)0.31, \\ 0.05\left(2\left(\dfrac{x-(1.2316-1.1)0.31}{(1.2316-1.1)0.31}\right)^2\right) \\ \text{for } (1.1658-1.1)0.31 \le x < (1.19-1.1)0.31, \\ \vdots \\ \dfrac{x+\frac{0.7414\cdot 0.31}{-0.31818}}{\frac{0.31}{-0.31818}} \\ \text{for } (3.21-1.1)0.31 \le x < (3.43-1.1)0.31, \\ \vdots \\ -0.03\left(1-2\left(\dfrac{x-(4.3-1.1)0.31}{(4.3-3.995)0.31}\right)^2\right) \\ \text{for } (4.1479-1.1)0.31 \le x < (4.3-1.1)0.31. \end{cases}$$

The mathematical tools used for polygons result in the creation of a common collection of curves representing the polygons over [0, 1]. Next, the selected elements of rough set theory will constitute a foundation for the classification of the curves.

## 7.5 The Classification of Letter-shaped Polygons

We return to the curves presented by Ex. 7.11 in order to accomplish their classification provided that we would like to determine their membership in the "*N*" class. The *y*-axis in Fig. 7.12 is divided in three regions. After analyzing the importance of the *y*-values we consider three intervals for them. The values of *y* belong to the interval (–0.3, 0.35) in the recognized case. Suppose that the *y*-values, occurring from –0.1 to 0.1 cannot provide us with essential information about the curve character and they are ignored. As a consequence, the code assigned to the *y*-value belonging to [–0.1, 0.1] is equal to 0. For decisive, positive *y*-values, the code of 1 is reserved while the negative *y*-values of a deterministic character obtain the code stated as –1.

Let us introduce the universe set $U = \{A^1, A^2, \ldots, A^n\}$ composed of continuous curves $A^1$, $A^2$, ..., $A^n$ approximating the polygons bearing the same names and representing different shapes of letters. The objects of *U* are determined by condition and decision attributes defined by the sets *B* and *D* respectively. We assume that the set *B* consists of sizes $x_k \in [0, 1]$, $k = 1, \ldots, m$, associated with values $code_{A^i}(x_k)$, $i = 1, \ldots, n$ that are equal to the integers –1, 0 and 1.

Since we want to assign some members to the "*N*" class, then set *D* obtains an attribute stated as "the membership of a polygon in "*N*"", where the membership is expressed as "*yes*", "*no*", "*unknown*".

The triple $I = (U, B, D)$ forms the decision table whose analysis generates the equivalence relation already introduced by (7.7), its classes given by (7.8) and two approximation sets of *X*, as recommended by (7.9) and (7.10). The relationship between class "*N*" and each member of *U* is estimated by (7.12).

### Example 7.14

We consider the data concerning $A^1$–$A^5$ and sampled in Fig. 7.10 as pictures of different letter-shaped cases. We decide $U = \{A^1, A^2, A^3, A^4, A^5\}$. The decision triple $I = (U, B, D)$ is expanded in Table 7.3. The objective of investigations is to revise the hypothesis formulated earlier in Ex. 7.11. As we remember, we have supposed that $A^1$, $A^3$ and $A^5$ fit the "*N*" class, $A^4$ resembles the letter "*W*", and we cannot strictly decide about the origin of $A^2$. Let us accomplish the appropriate rough classification by, at first, filling in some entry data in the mentioned decision table 7.3.

The table contains the values of condition and decision attributes.

Table 7.3: The decision table $I = (U, B, D)$ for letter-like curves $A^1$–$A^5$

| $A^i \backslash x_k$ | 0.125 | 0.250 | 0.375 | 0.500 | 0.625 | 0.750 | 0.875 | Class"$N$" |
|---|---|---|---|---|---|---|---|---|
| $A^1$ | 1 | 1 | 1 | 0 | −1 | −1 | 0 | *yes* |
| $A^2$ | 1 | 1 | 1 | 1 | 0 | 0 | −1 | *unknown* |
| $A^3$ | 0 | 1 | 1 | 1 | 0 | 0 | 0 | *yes* |
| $A^4$ | −1 | 0 | 0 | 1 | 0 | 0 | 0 | *no* |
| $A^5$ | 1 | 1 | 1 | 1 | 0 | 0 | −1 | *yes* |

The equivalence relation $I(B)$, provided in accordance with (7.7), is a set of pairs $I(B) = \{(A^1, A^1), (A^2, A^2), (A^3, A^3), (A^4, A^4), (A^5, A^5), (A^2, A^5), (A^5, A^2)\}$.

The equivalence classes of $I(B)$ are decided as the sets $IB(A^1) = \{A^1\}$, $IB(A^2) = \{A^2, A^5\}$, $IB(A^3) = \{A^3\}$, $IB(A^4) = \{A^4\}$, $IB(A^5) = \{A^2, A^5\}$ ·

The value of decision attribute "$N$" = "*yes*", generates the set $X = \{A^1, A^3, A^5\}$ that in turn is the most essential factor implementing sets $B_*(X) = \{A^1, A^3\}$, $B^*(X) = \{A^1, A^2, A^3, A^5\}$ and $B_{border}(X) = \{A^2, A^5\}$.

The polygon membership degrees, whose sizes confirm the membership in the "$N$" class, are obtained as:

$$\mu_{"N"}(A^1) = 1,\ \mu_{"N"}(A^2) = \frac{1}{2},\ \mu_{"N"}(A^3) = 1,\ \mu_{"N"}(A^4) = 0, \mu_{"N"}(A^5) = \frac{1}{2}.$$

By looking at the results of the accomplished analysis we can conclude that $A^1$ and $A^3$ are the true members of the "$N$" class in $U$, while $A^2$ and $A^5$ may belong to the investigated class to certain grades. The recognition of the curve nature aims at the special treatment of all sure and possible objects belonging to "$N$". We often know how to handle a class on the condition that its members are recognized.

Some finite sets of pairs are often interpolated by polygons that seldom have convenient equations mathematically expanded. Although there exists a large number of approximation methods applied to point sets, especially the different variations of least square regressions, we suggest applying a new procedure of approximation. This originates from the standard $\pi$ or $s$-functions in truncated forms that approximate the irregular parts of the polygons very smoothly.

The functions, called by us "the sampled, truncated $\pi$ ($s$)" are composed of the first and second degree-polynomials in the form of split definitions. The low degrees of approximating functions make further operations on them rather easy, which is an essential advantage of the method. One truncated $\pi$ or $s$-segment can approximate many nodes belonging to the point set that reduces a number of piecewise functions involved in the general definition of an approximating collection. But most of all we notice that "the sampled, truncated $\pi$ ($s$)" follows the changes of the polygon's pattern very sensitively, which guarantees the high thoroughness of approximation results.

A new process of approximation sometimes is invented in mathematics as an interesting theoretical item without greater practical validity. To prove the empirical aspect of "sampled truncated $\pi$ or $s$" we want to consider a classification praxis.

The accomplishment of a successful classification of unknown objects, possessing only some features typical of the considered class, is not an easy task. By applying rough set theory combined with earlier achievements in approximation, we could classify polygons within the same class even if they have an unknown origin. Two introduced sets, $B_*$ and $B^*$, act as a lower and an upper approximation of the investigated class. This makes it possible to assign its sure members and such ones that have most of the properties characteristic of the class. Moreover, we can easily exclude the polygons that do not satisfy the class's attributes.

If we need a pattern for another classification of objects obtained as some point sets, we can return to the discussed model and adapt it to other assumptions.

# References


1. Agadi, A., Penot, J-P.: A comparative Study of Various Notions of Approximation of Sets. J. of Approximation Theory, vol. 134, nr 1 (2005) 80-101
2. Adlassnig, K. P.: A Fuzzy Logical Model of Computer-assisted Medical Diagnosis. Methods of Information in Medicine 19, nr 3 (1980) 141-148
3. Adlassnig, K. P.: Fuzzy Modeling and Reasoning in a Medical Diagnostic Expert System. EVD in Medizin und Biologie 17, 1/2 (1986) 12-20
4. Bede, B., Nobuhara, H., Hirota, K.: Numerical Computation of Eigen Fuzzy Sets and Applications to Image Analysis. In: Dzitac, I., Maghiar, T., Popescu C. (eds.): Proc. of the International Conference on Computers and Communications, ICCC 2004. Univ. din Oradea, Romania (2004) 72-77
5. Baas, S. M., Kwakernaak, H.: Rating and Ranking of Multiple-aspect Alternatives Using Fuzzy Sets. Automatica, vol. 13, Pergamon Press (1977) 47-58
6. Barro, S., Marin, R. (eds.): Fuzzy Logic in Medicine. Studies in Fuzziness and Soft Computing Series, Springer-verlag, Berlin Heidelberg New York (2002)
7. Bouchon-Meunier, B.: Fuzzy Logic and Knowledge Representation Using Linguistic Modifiers. In: Zadeh, L. A., Kacprzyk, J. (eds.): Fuzzy Logic for the Management of Uncertainty, Wiley, New York (1992)
8. Belacel, N., Boulassel, M. R.: Multicriteria Fuzzy Assignment Method: a Useful Tool to Assist Medical Diagnosis. Artificial Intelligence in Medicine 21 (2001) 201-207
9. Bellman, R. E., Zadeh, L. A.: Decision Making in a Fuzzy Environment. Management Sci. Vol. 17, nr 4 (1970) 141-164
10. Blin, J. M., Whinston, A. B.: Fuzzy Sets and Social Choice. J. Cybern. Vol. 3 (1974) 28-36
11. Bortolan, G., Pedrycz, W.: An Interactive Framework for an Analysis of ECG Signals. Artificial Intelligence in Medicine 24 (2002) 109-132
12. Buckley, J., Eslami, E.: An Introduction to Fuzzy Logic and Fuzzy Sets. Advances in Soft Computing Series, Springer-verlag, Berlin Heidelberg New York (2002)
13. Carlsson, C., Fullér, R.: Benchmarking in Linguistic Importance Weighted Aggregations. Fuzzy Sets and Systems 114 (2000) 35-41
14. Carlsson, C., Fullér, R.: Fuzzy Reasoning in Decision Making and Optimization. Studies in Fuzziness and Soft Computing Series, Springer-Verlag, Berlin Heidelberg New York (2001)

15. Cherkassky, V., Gehring, D., Mulier, F.: Comparison of Adaptive Methods for Function Estimation for Samples. IEEE Transactions on Neural Networks, vol. 7, nr 4 (1996) 969-984
16. Chich-Hui Chiu, Wen-June Wang: A Simple Computation of MIN and MAX Operations for Fuzzy Numbers. Fuzzy Sets and Systems 126 (2002) 273-276
17. Cohen, M. E.: Comparative Approaches to Medical Reasoning. World Scientific, Singapore New Yersey Hong Kong (1995)
18. Detyniecki, M., Yager, R.: Ranking Fuzzy Numbers Using α-weighted Valuations. Internat. J. Uncertainty, Fuzziness Knowledge-Based Systems 8 (2000) 573-591
19. Dubois, D., Prade, H.: Fuzzy Real Algebra. Some Results. Fuzzy Sets and Systems 2 (1978) 327-348
20. Dubois, D., Prade, H.: Operations on Fuzzy Numbers. Int. J. Systems Sci., vol. 9, nr 6 (1978) 613-626
21. Dubois, D., Grabisch, M.: Modave, F., Prade, H.: Relating Decisions under Uncertainty and Multicriteria Decision Making Models. Int. J. of Intelligent Systems, vol. 15, nr 11 (2000) 967-979
22. Dug Hun Hong: Shape Preserving Multiplications of Fuzzy Numbers. Fuzzy Sets and Systems 123 (2001) 81-84
23. Facchinetti, G., Ghiselli Ricci, R., Muzziol, S.: Note of Ranking Fuzzy Triangular Numbers. Int. J. Intell. Syst. 13 (1998) 613-622
24. Fernández, M., Suárez, F., Gil, P.: T-eigen Fuzzy Sets, Inf. Sci. 75 (1993) 63-80
25. Fullér, R.: On Product-Sum of Triangular Fuzzy Numbers. Fuzzy Sets and Systems 41 (1991) 83-87
26. Fullér, R., Majlender, P.: On Weighted Possibilistic Mean and Variance of Fuzzy Numbers. Fuzzy Sets and Systems 136 (2003) 363-374
27. Gerstenkorn, T., Kurnatowska, A., Rakus, E.: The Application of Fuzzy Set Theory to Medical Diagnosis and Treatment of Inflammation of Genital Organs and Urinary tract in Women. Parasitological News, vol. 36, nr 5-6, Wrocław (1990) 251-267 (in Polish)
28. Gerstenkorn, T., Rakus, E.: On the Utility of the Notions of a Fuzzy Variable and a Linguistic Variable in Natural Science. Biometrical Letters, vol. 27, nr 1-2, Poznań (1990) 3-12 (in Polish)
29. Gerstenkorn, T., Rakus, E.: The Method of Calculating the Membership Degrees for Symptoms in Diagnostic Decisions. Cybernetics and Systems Research '92-Proceedings of the XI th European Meeting on Cybernetics and System Research, vol. 1, Vienna (1992) 479-486
30. Gerstenkorn, T., Rakus, E.: On Modelling Membership Function Values in Diagnostic Decisions. Biometrical Letters, vol. 3, nr 1, Poznań (1993) 3-12

31. Gerstenkorn, T., Rakus, E.: An Application of Fuzzy Set Theory to Differentiating the Effectiveness of Drugs in Treatment of Inflammation of Genital Organs. Fuzzy Sets and Systems 68 (1994) 327-333
32. Gerstenkorn, T., Rakus-Andersson, E.: Methods for Constructing Membership Functions in the Case when the Symptoms are Estimated Qualitatively and Quantitatively. Biocybernetics and Biomedical Engineering, vol 17, nr 1-2 (1997) 115-126
33. Ghaius, C.: Fuzzy Model and Control of a Fan-coil. Energy and Buildings 33 (2001) 545-551
34. Goetschel, R., Voxman, W.: Eigen Fuzzy Number Sets. Fuzzy Sets and Systems 16 (1985) 75-85
35. Haan, O.: A Free Algebraic Solution for the Planar Approximation. Nuclear Physics B 705 (2005) 563-575
36. Heilpern, S.: Representation and Application of Fuzzy Numbers. Fuzzy Sets and Systems 91 (1997) 259-268
37. Jacas, J., Recasens, J.: Fuzzy T-transitive Relations: Eigenvectors and Generators. Fuzzy Sets and Systems 72 (1995) 147-154
38. Jain, R.: Decision Making in the Presence of Fuzzy Variables. IEEE Trans. Syst. Man and Cybern. SMC-6 (1976) 698-703
39. Jain, R.: A Procedure for Multi-aspect Decision Making Using Fuzzy Sets. Int. J. Syst. Sci. 8 (1977) 1-7
40. Kacprzyk, J.: Zbiory rozmyte w analizie systemowej (Fuzzy Sets in System Analysis) PWN, Warszawa (1986) (in Polish)
41. Kaufmann, A., Gupta, M. M.: Introduction to Fuzzy Arithmetic Theory and Application. Van Nostrand Reinhold, New York (1991)
42. Kun-lun Zhang, Hirota K.: On Fuzzy Number Lattice. Fuzzy Sets and Systems 92 (1997) 113-122
43. Lavoué, G., Dupont, F., Baskurt, A.: A New Subdivision Based Approach for Piecewise Smooth Approximation of 3D Polygonal Curves. J. of Pattern Recognition Society, vol. 38, nr 8 (2005) 1139-1151
44. Lowen, R.: Fuzzy Set Theory: Basic Concepts, Techniques and Bibliography. Kluwer Academic Publishers, Dordrecht (1996)
45. Lucas, P.: Model-based Diagnosis in Medicine. Artificial Intelligence in Medicine 10 (1997) 201-208
46. Mesiar, R., Calvo, T., Yager, R. R.: Quantitative Weights and Aggregation. IEEE Transactions on Fuzzy Systems 12 (2004) 62-69
47. Mizumoto, M., Tanaka, K.: Some properties of Fuzzy Numbers. In: Gupta, M. M., Ragade, R. K., Yager, R. (eds.): Advances in Fuzzy Set Theory and Applications, North-Holland Publishing Company (1979)
48. Mordeson, J. N., Davender, S. M., Shih Chuang Cheng: Fuzzy Mathematics in Medicine. Studies in Fuzziness and Soft Computing Series, Springer-verlag, Berlin Heidelberg New York (2000)
49. Novák, V., Perfilieva, I.: Evaluating of Linguistic Expressions and Functional Fuzzy Theories in Fuzzy Logic. In: Zadeh, L. A., Kacprzyk, J.

(eds.): Computing with Words in Information – Intelligent Systems 2, vol. 33, Studies in Fuzziness and Soft Computing Series, Springer-verlag, Berlin Heidelberg New York (1999) 383-406

50. Pal, S. K., Mitra, P.: Case Generation Using Rough Sets with Fuzzy Representation. IEEE Transactions on Knowledge and Data Engineering, vol. 16, nr 3 (2004) 292-300
51. Pawlak, Z.: On Rough Sets. Bulletin of the EATCS 24 (1984) 94-108
52. Pawlak, Z.: Vagueness - a Rough Set View. Structures in Logic and Computer Science (1997) 106-117
53. Pawlak, Z.: Decision Networks. Proc. of Rough Sets and Current Trends in Computing 2004, Uppsala, Sweden (2004) 1-7
54. Pedrycz, W.: Fuzzy Sets Engineering, CRC Press, Boca Raton, FL (1995)
55. Pedrycz, W., Gomide, F.: An Introduction to Fuzzy Sets. Analysis and Design. MIT Press (1998)
56. Rakus, E.: Fuzzy Set Theory Assisting Medical Diagnosis and Appreciation of Drug Effectiveness. Doctor's dissertation, Medical Academy of Łódź (1991) (in Polish)
57. Rakus-Andersson, E., Gerstenkorn, T.: A Fuzzy Model of Decision Making to the Choice of a Medicine in the Case of Symptoms Prevailing after the Treatment. Bulletin of the Polish Academy of Sciences – Technical Sciences, vol. 45, nr 4 (1997) 633-641
58. Rakus-Andersson, E., Gerstenkorn T.: An Application of Fuzzy Set Theory in a Diagnostic Process Extended in Time. In: Trappl, R. (ed.): Proc. of the XIVth European Meeting on Cybernetics and System Research'98, vol. 1, University of Vienna and Austrian Society for Cybernetics Studies, Vienna (1998) 160-162
59. Rakus-Andersson, E.: A Fuzzy Decision Making Model Applied to the Choice of the Therapy in the Case of Symptoms not Disappearing after the Treatment. In: deBaets, B., Fodor, J., Kóczy, L. T. (eds.): Proc. of EUROFUSE-SIC'99, University of Veterinary Science – Department of Biomathematics and Informatics, Technical University of Budapest – Department of Telecommunications and Telematics, Budapest (1999) 298-303
60. Rakus-Andersson, E., Gerstenkorn T.: A Comparison of Different Fuzzy Decision Making Models Supporting the Optimal Therapy. In: Szczepaniak, P., Lisboa, P.J., Tsumoto, S. (eds.): Studies in Fuzziness and Soft Computing Series, Springer-verlag, Berlin Heidelberg New York (1999) 561-572
61. Rakus-Andersson, E., Gerstenkorn, T.: A Diagnostic Process Extended in Time as a Fuzzy Model. In: Dubois, D. (ed.): Computing Anticipatory Systems. Casys'98 – Second International Conference, American Institute of Physics, Woodbury, New York (1999) 283-288
62. Rakus-Andersson, E.: A Fuzzy Group-Decision Making Model Applied to the Choice of the Optimal Medicine in the Case of Symptoms not Disappearing after the Treatment. In: Dubois, D. (ed.): The International

Journal of Computing Anticipatory Systems, University of Liège, Chaos, Liège (1999) 141-152
63. Rakus-Andersson, E.: The Newton Interpolation Method with Fuzzy Numbers as the Entries. In: Rutkowski, L., Kacprzyk J. (eds.): Neural Networks and Soft Computing, Proc. of the Sixth International Conference on Neural Network and Soft Computing, Studies in Fuzziness and Soft Computing Series, Springer-verlag, Berlin Heidelberg New York (2003) 310-315
64. Rakus-Andersson, E.: An Application of Fuzzy Numbers in Eigen Fuzzy Set Problem to Differentiating the Effectiveness of Drugs. In: Yinming Liu, Guoqing Chen (eds.): Proc. of the International Conference on Fuzzy Information Processing – Theories and Applications, Tsinghua University Press – Springer (2003) 85-90
65. Rakus-Andersson, E., Salomonsson, M.: The Truncated $\pi$-functions in Approximation of Multi-shaped Polygons. In: deBeats, B., de Caluwe, R., de Tre, G., Fodor, J., Kacprzyk, J., Zadrożny, S. (eds.): Current Issues in Data and Knowledge Engineering, Proc. of EUROFUSE 2004 – EURO WG on Fuzzy Sets, Exit, Warsaw (2004) 444-452
66. Rakus-Andersson, E., Salomonsson, M.: $\Pi$-truncated Functions and Rough Sets in the Classification of Internet Protocols. In: Yingming Liu, Guoqing Chen, Mingsheng Ying (eds.): Proc. of Eleventh International Fuzzy Systems Association World Congress – IFSA 2005, Beijing, Tsinghua University Press – Springer (2005) 1487-1492
67. Rakus-Andersson, E.: *S*-truncated Functions and Rough Sets in Approximation and Classification of Polygons. Proc. of Modeling Decisions for Artificial Intelligence – MDAI 2005, Tsukuba, CD-ROM, paper nr 049, Consejo Superior de Investigaciones Cientificas (2005)
68. Saaty, T. L.: Exploring the Interface Between Hierarchies, Multiplied Objectives and Fuzzy Sets. Fuzzy Sets and Systems 1 (1978) 57-68
69. Sadegh-Zadeh, K.: The Fuzzy Revolution: Goodbye to the Aristotelian Weltanschauung. Artificial Intelligence in Medicine 21 (2000) 1-25
70. Saitta, L., Torasso, P.: Fuzzy Characterization of Coronary Disease. Fuzzy Sets and Systems 5 (1981) 245-258
71. Salmeri, M., Mencattini, A., Rovatti, R.: Function Approximation Using Non-normalized SISO Fuzzy Systems. International Journal of Approximate Reasoning 26 (2001) 211-231
72. Sanchez, E.: Resolution of Eigen Fuzzy Set Equations. Fuzzy Sets and Systems 1 (1978) 69-74
73. Sanchez, E.: Eigen Fuzzy Sets and Fuzzy Relations. Journal of Mathematical Analysis and Applications 81 (1981) 399-421
74. Sanchez, E.: Truth Qualification and Fuzzy Relations in Natural Languages, Application to Medical Diagnosis. Fuzzy Sets and Systems 84 (1996) 155-167

75. Schmitt, M., Teodorescu, H. N., Jain, A.: Computational Intelligence Processing in Medical Diagnosis. Studies in Fuzziness and Soft Computing Series, Springer-verlag, Berlin Heidelberg New York (2002)
76. Steimann, F., Adlassnig, K. P.: Clinical Monitoring with Fuzzy Automata. Fuzzy Sets and Systems 61 (1994) 37-42
77. Steimann, F., Adlassnig, K. P.: Fuzzy Medical Diagnosis. In: Ruspini, E., Bonissone, P., Pedrycz, W. (eds.): Handbook of Fuzzy Computation, Institute of Physics Publishing, Bristol Philadelphia (1998) G13.1:1-G13.1:14
78. Wagenknecht, M., Hartmann, K.: On the Construction of Fuzzy Eigen Solutions in Given Regions. Fuzzy Sets and Systems 20 (1986) 55-65
79. Wang, X., Kerre, E.: Reasonable Properties for the Ordering of Fuzzy Quantities (I), (II). Fuzzy Sets and Systems 118 (2001) 375-385, 387-405
80. Yager, R. R.: Multiple Objective Decision-Making Using Fuzzy Sets. Int. J. Man-Machine Studies 9 (1977) 375-382
81. Yager, R. R.: Fuzzy Decision Making Including Unequal Objectives. Fuzzy Sets and Systems 1 (1978) 87-95
82. Yager, R. R., Kacprzyk, J.: The Ordered Weighted Averaging Operators: Theory and Applications. Kluwer, Norwell, MA (1997)
83. Yager, R. R.: Modeling Uncertainty Using Partial Information. Inf. Sci. vol. 121 (1999) 271-294
84. Yager, R. R.: Decision Making Using Minimization of Regret. Int. J. of Approximate Reasoning 36 (2004) 109-128
85. Yager, R. R.: Uncertainty Modeling and Decision Support. Reliability Engineering and System Safety, vol. 85 (2004) 341-354
86. Yager, R. R.: Generalized OWA Aggregation Operators. Fuzzy Optimization and Decision Making 3 (2004) 93-107
87. Yao Janis Fan-Fang, Yao Jing-Shing: Fuzzy Decision Making for Medical Diagnosis Based on Fuzzy Number and Compositional Rule of Inference. Fuzzy Sets and Systems 120 (2001) 351-366
88. Zadeh, L. A.: Fuzzy sets. Inf. Control 8 (1965) 338-353
89. Zadeh, L. A.: Outline of a New Approach to the Analysis of Complex Systems and Decision Processes. IEEE Trans. Systems, Man Cybernet. 3 (1973) 28-48
90. Zadeh, L. A.: The Concept of a Linguistic Variable and its Application to Approximate Reasoning. Inf. Sci. 8 (1975) 199-249
91. Zadeh, L. A.: Calculus of Fuzzy Restrictions. Fuzzy Sets and Their Applications to Cognitive and Decision Processes. Academic Press, London (1975)
92. Zadeh, L. A.: A Computational Approach to Fuzzy Quantifiers in Natural Languages. Computers and Mathematics 9 (1983) 149-184
93. Zadeh, L. A.: Test-score Semantics as a Basis for a Computational Approach to the Representation of Meaning. Literary and Linguistic Computing 1 (1986) 24-35

94. Zadeh, L. A.: From Computing with Numbers to Computing with Words – From Manipulation of Measurements to Manipulation of Perceptions. IEEE Transactions on Circuits and Systems 45 (1999) 105-119
95. Zimmermann, H. J.: Fuzzy Set Theory and Its Applications. 3rd edn, Kluwer Academic Publishers, Boston (1996)

# Index

accuracy of approximation, 89
$\alpha$-level of a fuzzy set, 141
atomic expression, 46, 120

boundary set, 89, 167
bounded norm, 18

cardinality of a set, 89
Cartesian product, 17, 23
characteristic equation, 150
characteristic function, 4
clock-like polygons, 155, 156
compatibility degree, 19
complement of a fuzzy set, 14, 15
compound qualitative feature, 33, 34, 35
composition of relations, 25
  max-av, 28, 29
  max-min, 26, 33, 55, 56, 57, 94, 115, 123
  max-prod, 28
concentration operator, 42
crisp set, 5
criteria-objectives, 145, 148

decision attribute, 88, 166, 179,
decision space, 126
decisive character of symptom for diagnosis, 45, 50, 51, 52, 82
diagnostic process extended in time, 80
dilution operator, 42
distance between fuzzy sets, 71, 72, 75, 76, 78, 85
double negation law, 56
drug effectiveness level, 102, 123

eigen fuzzy set, 94, 97, 117
eigen value of a matrix, 150
eigen vector of a matrix, 150
elementary set, 87, 88
equivalence class, 88, 166, 180
equivalence relation, 88, 166, 179

finite set, 4
fuzzy constraint, 19, 131
fuzzy number in the *L–R* form, 104, 109, 119
fuzzy relation, 23, 24, 34, 54, 58, 59, 66, 67, 68, 69, 81, 82, 83, 94, 96, 98, 100, 101, 102, 119
fuzzy set, 5, 11, 13, 14, 72, 73, 76, 84, 85, 95, 131, 132, 133, 134, 135, 145
fuzzy set of type-1, 116
fuzzy set of type-2, 116, 117, 124
fuzzy utility, 128, 135
fuzzy variable, 19, 45, 46

greatest eigen fuzzy set, 96
greatest eigen fuzzy set with fuzzy numbers, 117, 118
group order relation, 140

hedge, 48

inclusion of fuzzy sets, 94, 95
indiscernibility relation, 87, 166
infinite set, 4
intersection of fuzzy sets, 14

Jain's operator, 133

largest norm, 18
least eigen fuzzy set, 97, 98
letter-like polygons, 168, 169
linguistic variable, 21, 34, 35, 129
lower approximation, 89, 166

matrix, 24
maximum for two fuzzy numbers, 107, 111, 112

medical knowledge, 53, 82
membership degree, 5, 89, 100, 118, 121, 122, 135, 140, 148, 167
membership function, 5, 37, 41, 47, 48, 49, 50, 55, 56, 57, 65, 66, 67, 81, 82, 94, 104, 115, 117, 119, 130,148
minimum decision rule, 148
minimum for two fuzzy numbers, 106, 109
minimum norm, 18
minimization of regret, 152
modus ponens law, 32, 55, 82
modus tollens law, 54, 56, 83
multiplication of matrices, 25, 26

optimal decision, 135, 148
OWA operator, 63, 64, 66, 70, 121, 122

patient – diagnosis relation, 32, 55
patient – symptom relation, 31, 33
payoff matrix, 152
$\pi$-function, 9, 157, 158
point set, 155
polygon, 155
presence of the symptom in diagnosis, 22, 45, 50, 51, 52, 82

quantitative feature, 33, 40, 41

reference functions, 104
reflexive relation, 88
regret matrix, 152, 153
rough set, 87, 165,

sampled truncated $\pi$, 157, 164, 167
sampled truncated $s$, 169, 172
set of condition attributes, 87, 166, 179
set of diagnoses, 31, 81
set of patients, 31, 87
set of physicians, 140
set of stages of observations, 81
set of symptoms, 31, 81, 87, 119
$s$-function, 8, 36, 170
$s$-norm, 18
simple qualitative feature, 33, 34
space of $L$-$R$ fuzzy numbers, 104
space of states-results, 127
stage – diagnosis relation, 82, 84
stage – symptom relation, 81
support of a fuzzy set, 5, 119
symmetric relation, 88
symptom – diagnosis relation, 31, 32, 45

$t$-norm, 17, 18
total acceptance of diagnosis, 85
total order, 142
total rejection of diagnosis, 85
transitive relation, 88
truncated $\pi$-function, 161
truncated $s$-function, 172

union of crisp sets, 12
union of fuzzy sets, 13
universe set, 87, 166, 179
upper approximation, 89, 166
utility matrix, 128

weights of answers, 35
weights of criteria-objectives, 148, 150, 153
weights of symptoms, 122

# Elisabeth Rakus-Andersson
# Fuzzy and Rough Techniques in Medical Models and Medication
# The back page

This volume provides readers with selected fuzzy and rough tools used to medical tasks, especially diagnosing and medication. To build a link between theoretical, mathematical excerpts and practical medical applications, the contents is formed as a sequence of occurrences in which a patient appears to be diagnosed and cured. The fuzzy and rough elements are inserted in the book in the order required by the presentation of medical substance to maintain the logical unity of the book's essence.

In conformity with this pattern the essay presents in turn some necessary elements of fuzzy set theory, the classical fuzzy diagnostic model with extensions, the fuzzy diagnostic model with clinical examinations extended throughout time based on distance theory, methods of drug effectiveness measurements and algorithms selecting the optimal medicine. As the complement, the solution of an approximation problem is suggested to find a curve that surrounds two-dimensional clock-like point sets with the little approximation error.

A lot of appealing examples are added to facilitate comprehension of theoretical principles for a reader, so that even a beginner in fuzzy set theory can follow calculation steps without implementing computer programs. It should be emphasized that all models are also applicable to other fields, especially to technical domains after necessary adaptations. This confirms the existence of the large spectrum of applicable fuzzy and rough methods not only in medicine but also in natural sciences.

Printed in the United States
70762LV00002B/337-360

9 783540 497073